Career Planning for Psychiatrists

ISSUES IN PSYCHIATRY

Joseph D. Bloom, M.D.
Series Editor

Career Planning for Psychiatrists

Edited by

Kathleen M. Mogul, M.D.
and
Leah J. Dickstein, M.D.

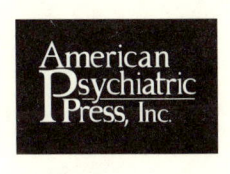

American Psychiatric Press, Inc.

Washington, DC
London, England

Note: The authors have worked to ensure that all information in this book concerning drug dosages, schedules, and routes of administration is accurate as of the time of publication and consistent with standards set by the U.S. Food and Drug Administration and the general medical community. As medical research and practice advance, however, therapeutic standards may change. For this reason and because human and mechanical errors sometimes occur, we recommend that readers follow the advice of a physician who is directly involved in their care or the care of a member of their family.

Books published by the American Psychiatric Press, Inc., represent the views and opinions of the individual authors and do not necessarily represent the policies and opinions of the Press or the American Psychiatric Association.

Copyright © 1995 American Psychiatric Press, Inc.
ALL RIGHTS RESERVED
Manufactured in the United States of America on acid-free paper
98 97 96 95   4 3 2 1
First Edition
American Psychiatric Press, Inc.
1400 K Street, N.W., Washington, DC 20005

Library of Congress Cataloging-in-Publication Data
Career planning for psychiatrists /edited by Kathleen M. Mogul, Leah J. Dickstein. — 1st ed.
    p.   cm. — (Issues in psychiatry)
  Includes bibliographical references and index.
  ISBN 0-88048-197-8
  1. Psychiatry—Vocational guidance. 2. Psychiatry—Practice.
I. Mogul, Kathleen M., 1927- . II. Dickstein, Leah J., 1934- . III. Series.
  [DNLM: 1. Psychiatry. 2. Career Mobility. 3. Professional Practice. 4. Specialties, Medical.   WM 21 C2713 1995]
  RC440.8.C37   1995
  616.89′023—dc20
  DNLM/DLC   95-1384
  for Library of Congress   CIP

British Library Cataloguing in Publication Data
A CIP record is available from the British Library.

Contents

Contributors ix

History and Acknowledgments xv

Foreword xvii
Stephen C. Scheiber, M.D.

Introduction xxi
Kathleen M. Mogul, M.D., and Leah J. Dickstein, M.D.

Section I: Research and Frontiers in Psychiatry

CHAPTER ONE

Psychiatric Research 3
Harold Alan Pincus, M.D.

CHAPTER TWO

Zen and the Art of Biological Psychiatry Research 17
John M. Morihisa, M.D.

CHAPTER THREE

Psychopharmacology 25
George W. Arana, M.D., and Laura Rames, M.D.

CHAPTER FOUR

Sleep Disorders Medicine (Somnology) 35
Milton Kramer, M.D.

Section II: Setting-Related Careers
Hospital-Based Practice

CHAPTER FIVE

Inpatient Psychiatry 51
Margaret J. Dorfman, M.D., and John J. Haggerty, Jr., M.D.

CHAPTER SIX

Emergency Psychiatry 65
Gail M. Barton, M.D., M.P.H.

CHAPTER SEVEN

Consultation-Liaison Psychiatry 77
Thomas N. Wise, M.D., and Miriam B. Rosenthal, M.D.

Outpatient-Based Practice

CHAPTER EIGHT

Private Practice 91
Kathleen M. Mogul, M.D., and Joseph E. V. Rubin, M.D.

CHAPTER NINE

Psychiatric Practice in Industry 103
David B. Robbins, M.D., M.P.H.

CHAPTER TEN

**Psychiatric Practice in College and
University Mental Health Services** 113
Leah J. Dickstein, M.D.

Organized Care Practice

CHAPTER ELEVEN

Health Maintenance Organization Psychiatry 125
  Judith L. Feldman, M.D.

CHAPTER TWELVE

Community Psychiatry 133
  Gordon H. Clark, Jr., M.D.

CHAPTER THIRTEEN

Military Psychiatry 143
  Maria E. Esposito, M.D., and Robert J. Ursano, M.D.

Academic Psychiatry

CHAPTER FOURTEEN

Academic Psychiatry 157
  Leah J. Dickstein, M.D.

Section III: Administrative Psychiatry

CHAPTER FIFTEEN

Administrative Psychiatry 171
  Carolyn B. Robinowitz, M.D.

Section IV: Practice by Specialty Area
Focus on Unique Populations

CHAPTER SIXTEEN

Child Psychiatry 185
  Helen R. Beiser, M.D., and Benjamin Garber, M.D.

CHAPTER SEVENTEEN

Geriatric Psychiatry 197
    Marion Z. Goldstein, M.D., and Kye Kim, M.D.

CHAPTER EIGHTEEN

Forensic Psychiatry 211
    Naomi Goldstein, M.D., and Thomas G. Gutheil, M.D.

CHAPTER NINETEEN

Addiction Psychiatry 227
    Sheila B. Blume, M.D.

Focus on Specific Treatment Modalities

CHAPTER TWENTY

Psychoanalysis 243
    Malkah T. Notman, M.D.

CHAPTER TWENTY-ONE

Family Therapy 255
    Joan J. Zilbach, M.D.

CHAPTER TWENTY-TWO

Group Therapy 261
    Marcia Slomowitz, M.D.

Conclusion 269
    Leah J. Dickstein, M.D., and Kathleen M. Mogul, M.D.

Index 273

Contributors

George W. Arana, M.D.
Executive Medical Director, Medical University of South Carolina, Medical Center, Charleston, South Carolina

Gail M. Barton, M.D., M.P.H.
Professor of Psychiatry, Dartmouth Medical School, Hanover, New Hampshire; Director of Mental Hygiene, Veterans Administration Hospital, White River Junction, Vermont

Helen R. Beiser, M.D.
Clinical Professor of Psychiatry, Emeritus, University of Illinois College of Medicine, Chicago, Illinois; Training and Supervising Analyst, Emeritus, Institute for Psychoanalysis, Chicago, Illinois

Sheila B. Blume, M.D.
Medical Director, Alcoholism, Chemical Dependency, and Compulsive Gambling Programs, South Oaks Hospital, Amityville, New York; Clinical Professor of Psychiatry, State University of New York at Stony Brook, New York

Gordon H. Clark, Jr., M.D.
Clinical Assistant Professor of Psychiatry, University of Pittsburgh School of Medicine, Pittsburgh, Pennsylvania; Medical Advisor, Deerfield Management Group, Erie, Pennsylvania; Founding President, American Association of Community Psychiatrists

Leah J. Dickstein, M.D.
Professor, Department of Psychiatry and Behavioral Sciences; Associate Chair for Academic Affairs; and Associate Dean for Faculty and Student Advocacy, University of Louisville School of Medicine, Louisville, Kentucky

Margaret J. Dorfman, M.D.
Chief, Mental Health Department, Kaiser Permanente—Durham/Chapel Hill Service Area, Chapel Hill, North Carolina

Maria E. Esposito, M.D.
Colonel, Military Corps, U. S. Army; Director, Residency Training, Walter Reed Army Medical Center, Washington, DC; Assistant Professor, Department of Psychiatry, Uniformed Services University of the Health Sciences, Bethesda, Maryland

Judith L. Feldman, M.D.
Associate Chief, Central Psychiatric Programs, Harvard Community Health Plan, Miner Street Treatment Center, Boston, Massachusetts; Clinical Instructor in Psychiatry, Harvard Medical School, Boston, Massachusetts

Benjamin Garber, M.D.
Director, Barr-Harris Center for the Study of Parent Loss, Chicago, Illinois; Training and Supervising Analyst, Institute for Psychoanalysis, Chicago, Illinois

Marion Zucker Goldstein, M.D.
Chief, Geriatric Psychiatry Inpatient Unit, and Director, Division of Geriatric Psychiatry, Erie County Medical Center, Buffalo, New York; Clinical Associate Professor, Department of Psychiatry and Internal Medicine, School of Medicine and Biomedical Sciences, State University of New York at Buffalo, New York

Naomi Goldstein, M.D.
Clinical Professor of Psychiatry, New York University Medical School, New York, New York

Thomas G. Gutheil, M.D.
Professor of Psychiatry, Co-Director of the Program in Psychiatry and the Law, Harvard Medical School, Boston, Massachusetts

Contributors

John J. Haggerty, Jr., M.D.
Associate Professor, Department of Psychiatry, University of North Carolina School of Medicine at Chapel Hill, North Carolina

Kye Kim, M.D.
Chief, Geriatric Psychiatry Inpatient Unit, Buffalo Veterans Administration Medical Center, Buffalo, New York; Clinical Assistant Professor, Department of Psychiatry, School of Medicine and Biomedical Sciences, State University of New York at Buffalo, New York

Milton Kramer, M.D.
Director, Sleep Disorders Center, Bethesda Oak Hospital, Cincinnati, Ohio; Professor, University of Cincinnati, Departments of Psychiatry and Psychology, Cincinnati, Ohio; Clinical Professor of Psychiatry, Wright State University, Dayton, Ohio

Kathleen M. Mogul, M.D.
Associate Clinical Professor of Psychiatry, Tufts University Medical School, Newton, Massachusetts

John M. Morihisa, M.D.
Professor and Chairman, Department of Psychiatry, Albany Medical College, Albany, New York

Malkah T. Notman, M.D.
Acting Chairperson, Department of Psychiatry, The Cambridge Hospital; Clinical Professor of Psychiatry, Harvard Medical School, Cambridge, Massachusetts; Training and Supervising Psychoanalyst, Boston Psychoanalytic Institute, Boston, Massachusetts

Harold Alan Pincus, M.D.
Deputy Medical Director, Director of Office of Research, American Psychiatric Association, Washington, DC; Clinical Professor, Department of Psychiatry and Behavioral Sciences, George Washington University, Washington, DC

Laura Rames, M.D.
Assistant Professor in Psychiatry, Department of Psychiatry and Behavioral Sciences, Medical University of South Carolina, Charleston; Attending Physician, Charleston Memorial Hospital Psychiatric Unit

David B. Robbins, M.D., M.P.H.
Associate Clinical Professor, Department of Psychiatry, New York Medical College, Chappaqua, New York

Carolyn B. Robinowitz, M.D.
Associate Dean of Students and Professor of Psychiatry, Georgetown University School of Medicine, Washington, DC; former Senior Deputy Medical Director, American Psychiatric Association, Washington, DC

Miriam B. Rosenthal, M.D.
Associate Professor, Psychiatry and Reproductive Biology, Case Western Reserve University, Cleveland, Ohio; Chief of Behavioral Medicine, Department of Obstetrics/Gynecology, Macdonald University Women's Hospital, Cleveland, Ohio

Joseph E. V. Rubin, M.D.
Private practice in psychiatry, Portland, Maine

Marcia Slomowitz, M.D.
Assistant Professor of Psychiatry, Department of Psychiatry and Behavioral Sciences, Northwestern University Medical School, Chicago, Illinois; Director, Inpatient Psychiatry, Northwestern Memorial Hospital, Chicago, Illinois

Robert J. Ursano, M.D.
Professor and Chairman, Department of Psychiatry, Uniformed Services University of the Health Sciences, Bethesda, Maryland

Thomas N. Wise, M.D.
Professor and Vice-Chairman, Department of Psychiatry, Georgetown University, Washington, DC; Chairman, Department of Psychiatry, Fairfax Hospital, Falls Church, Virginia

Joan J. Zilbach, M.D.
Faculty, Training, and Supervising Analyst, Boston Psychoanalytic Institute, Boston, Massachusetts; Professor and Regional Senior Faculty, Fielding Institute, Santa Barbara, California

History and Acknowledgments

This book started with a course entitled "Special Issues for Women Psychiatrists in Planning and Managing a Career in the 80s," presented at the scientific meetings held during the 1987 American Psychiatric Association annual meeting. One of the editors (KMM) originally proposed the course and both editors (KMM and LJD) participated in the course as faculty. American Psychiatric Press, Inc. (APPI), contacted the editors to expand the course into a book. Upon submission of the chapters, APPI editors decided that the book was of sufficient general interest to warrant revision and expansion to include the needs of male as well as female psychiatrists. Thus, finally, after a long and arduous gestation, the current book evolved.

We wish to thank the editors at APPI who helped with the evolution of the book, particularly Dr. Judith Gold for her original interest; Dr. Carol Nadelson for her support and helpful suggestions; and Dr. Joseph Bloom, editor of the Issues in Psychiatry series, whose careful, critical reading and suggestions helped sharpen the focus of the book. We appreciate the editorial contribution and help of Rebecca Richters, Project Editor, and others on the APPI staff. Most of all, we thank the authors who wrote and patiently rewrote chapters. Finally, we thank our families who supported us and benignly tolerated many hours of editing at our desks and over the telephone. It is to them that we dedicate this book.

Foreword

Stephen C. Scheiber, M.D.[*]

This book's topic has relevance for a diverse group of readers—from medical students considering a career in psychiatry, to faculty advisers assisting students in career development, to practitioners in other medical specialties interested in what psychiatry has to offer, including those thinking of switching to psychiatry as a career. Especially timely is the editors' sensitivity to and focus on the opportunities that psychiatry holds for women and other minority groups, including international medical students.

All recognized leaders in their respective fields, the chapter authors not only provide enthusiastic endorsements of their respective areas of practice but also communicate their enormous respect for the scope and complexity of the subject matter. In addition, their frank and open assessments of the pros and cons of their respective specialties provide valuable information that should enable those considering careers in these practice areas to make informed decisions.

The multiplicity of the perspectives presented by the authors should also help correct many of the negative and stereotypic views of psychiatry prevalent in media portrayals of the profession and its practitioners. Among the myths that this book should be useful in dispelling is the view of psychiatry as monolithic and monothematic. The reality is far otherwise, as the authors demonstrate. The great diversity of the field—a diversity that carries with it a multitude of opportunities for individuals of many different interests and backgrounds—is evident in the breadth of topics covered in this volume.

In the book's first section, Research and Frontiers in Psychiatry, the authors enumerate the recent exciting advances in the field, from the revolutionary strides in psychopharmacology to the unraveling of the mysteries of sleep. Their enthusiasm for and obvious dedication to

---
[*] Executive Vice President, American Board of Psychiatry and Neurology.

their work infuse these chapters with a sense of the exhilaration inherent in participating in the search for new meanings of human behavior.

In the next two sections, Setting-Related Careers and Administrative Psychiatry, the authors demonstrate how clinical knowledge is integrated and applied in a variety of settings: hospital inpatient, general medical, nonpsychiatric wards, and outpatient environments. Also addressed are the opportunities in structured settings, such as the community, the military, and the managed care arena. Of special potential benefit to the reader are the contributors' insights regarding the advantages and disadvantages of these environments and their thoughts about how work in them can be balanced with personal considerations. I particularly commend to the reader Dickstein's chapter on Academic Psychiatry, which describes in depth the application of clinical skills with a specific population, and Robinowitz's chapter on Administrative Psychiatry, which establishes the importance of a clinical base even in performance of largely nonclinical work.

The fourth section—Specialty Areas—contains chapters on unique populations, first focusing on careers with patients at the extremes of the life cycle (children, adolescents, and the elderly); then on subspecialties such as addiction psychiatry and forensic psychiatry (both of which are recognized subspecialties of the American Board of Psychiatry and Neurology); and finally on specific modalities (psychoanalysis and family and group therapies).

I write this foreword as someone who cares about attracting medical students and practitioners from other specialties into the field of psychiatry. Dedicated, talented, and enthusiastic individuals are needed to continue the vital work of this century's psychiatrists—to make valuable contributions and to receive tremendous personal and professional satisfaction in return. Psychiatry in its many career manifestations—clinical settings, target populations, therapeutic modalities, and specialties—offers a rich array of opportunities and options. For those contemplating these choices, the stimulating and thought-provoking discussions in this book provide all of the necessary ingredients for career decision-making.

Introduction

Kathleen M. Mogul, M.D., and Leah J. Dickstein, M.D.

This book presents a menu of career possibilities for those who are confronting decisions about psychiatry as a specialty and choices about their work within this specialty.

To medical students, we wish to give a taste of the diversity and rich opportunities available in the field of psychiatry. To them as well as psychiatric residents, we wish to present the many settings in which psychiatrists practice, and the different degrees of specialized expertise that can be acquired and used in both the biological and the psychosocial realms. We hope to present a menu that provides the essential ingredients and qualities of each offering and conveys that it is possible either to select one "item" only or, as is more commonly done, to combine different options either simultaneously or sequentially. In keeping with the latter option, we hope this book provides some help to practicing psychiatrists who wish to add new skills to their existing ones, to further subspecialize, or to change practice settings. Although this book can certainly be sampled by selective, topical reading, we urge readers to read the whole book so that they might gain a more comprehensive view of what a psychiatric career might offer and what combinations might be considered.

In making career plans, particularly in the 1990s and possibly in psychiatry more than in other medical specialties, it is difficult to predict with certainty what one may want to do as time goes on. It is important to think ahead, consider different options, and position oneself as well as possible for the present as well as for the future.

We think of career plans to be made in a matrix of different trajectories or time lines, each of which is largely independent of the others and predictable only to a limited degree. In this introduction we cover the four trajectories that we feel most strongly affect the career choices a psychiatrist will follow, the first two of which are beyond the control of the individual practitioner and the last two of which are more firmly in the practitioner's control: 1) changes in psychiatric practice, 2) changes in the health care delivery system, 3) personal time lines, and 4) family time lines.

Changes in Psychiatric Practice

One must consider first where psychiatry is going and how it is changing. Just as psychoactive medicines barely existed 30 years ago, and have changed and continue to change the practice of psychiatry in every setting, so it is hard to know what further advances in neurochemistry, psychoneuroimmunology, and genetics and in diagnostic and treatment modalities await us. It is clear, however, that there will be many more undreamed-of advances, that the possibilities lend excitement to psychiatric research, and that changes will continuously affect the way psychiatrists treat patients.

Emergence of new subspecialties. Although the incidence of some psychiatric illnesses remains remarkably steady, new diagnostic approaches have changed the perceived incidence of others; there have also been changes in illness patterns over the years that reveal different or new clinical needs. Changes in population patterns in the incidence of some conditions, and in clinical perspectives, have defined new areas of research and practice, leading to increased expertise and areas of subspecialization in psychiatry. Geriatric practice and the field of chemical dependency disorders continue to grow. Only recently has psychiatric attention begun to focus on those who have experienced trauma and abuse. New methods of dealing with infertility have produced not only new solutions to problems with fertility but also new kinds of emotional problems for the affected adults and children. A new illness, acquired immunodeficiency syndrome (AIDS), with its primary and secondary psychiatric effects, has led to new demands on psychiatrists that are only gradually becoming evident, but whose extent cannot even be guessed.

Remedicalization of psychiatry. Other tensions, unsettled issues, and possible trends affect the field of psychiatry and deserve consideration by those choosing a career path in this specialty. Many factors—research into the biological bases of mental disorders and in psychopharmacology, economic and health care delivery considerations, and psychiatrists' desire for a secure and clear professional identity—have led to what is referred to as the *remedicalization* of psychiatry. Although this change in emphasis has stemmed from progress in researching etiologies of psychiatric illnesses and offers many new opportunities for psychiatrists, it has also had negative effects within psychiatry, kindling a growing concern that psychiatry is "losing the mind" (Reiser 1988) as it gains the brain. Whereas in the past, psychiatry department chairs were often psychoanalysts and training programs offered residents a thorough grounding in the theories and practice of psychotherapy, many departments are now headed by psychiatrist-researchers who have little interest in or respect for the psychosocial aspects of psychiatry; consequently, too many training programs offer little more than lip service to training in these aspects of the field. We see this development as a loss to psychiatry, psychiatrists, and, mainly, psychiatric patients, as we continue to consider the unique contribution of psychiatry the integration of the biological with the psychosocial. We are pleased that the authors of the chapters on research and biological aspects of psychiatry in this book all stress the primacy of the clinical psychological experience in training.

Psychiatrists' lack of exclusivity as psychotherapists. A related question is, Who should do psychotherapy? Economic and other factors currently tend to press psychiatrists into performing only those services for which they alone, among mental health professionals, are qualified—namely, diagnosing psychiatric disorders and prescribing medication. Many, though not all, psychiatrists continue to believe that well-trained psychiatrists are uniquely qualified to offer the combination of descriptive, social, and psychodynamic diagnoses for patients and the ensuing combination of psychotherapeutic and psychopharmacological treatments. Often physicians specialize in psychiatry because they are interested in people's problems, conflicts, thoughts, and feelings and the interrelation between these elements and patients' illnesses, treatment responses, and recovery. These psychiatrists want to offer psychotherapy among their skilled services. How individual psychiatrists in the 1990s and beyond resolve this will depend on a combination of the variables in psychotherapy, including the efficacy of psychotherapy, and opportunities in the health care system.

Subspecialization. As in other fields of medicine, in psychiatry there is a move toward greater specialization. In 1989, the American Psychiatric Association developed criteria for the acceptance of groups as subspecialties, whereby members who meet certain criteria related to training, experience, and examination in a subspecialty, and who have received previous certification in general psychiatry, can qualify for "added qualifications" from the American Board of Psychiatry and Neurology (ABPN). Geriatric psychiatry and the field of substance addiction and abuse are two areas of practice that have been approved as subspecialties on the basis of these criteria; other groups are in the process of applying for this status. (Child psychiatry has been a subspecialty for many years, whereas forensic and administrative psychiatry have developed their own subspecialty criteria without the involvement of the ABPN.)

Given this trend toward subspecialization, and even the practice of less formally recognized specialties defined by diagnostic category (e.g., eating disorders, posttraumatic stress disorder, depression), many psychiatrists are concerned that the field of psychiatry will be carved up into many specialties with decreased demand for and acceptance of generalists, although at times, generalists may be those best able to offer the most appropriate care in complex clinical situations. Once again, a combination of outside forces and individual predilections will determine whether a particular psychiatrist elects to remain a generalist, develops an added interest and expertise in one or more areas, or opts to specialize entirely.

Changes in the Health Care Delivery System

The changes in the ways that health care is delivered constitute a second "trajectory." Realities and predictions about the economics and systems of health care delivery change so rapidly that there will most likely be several changes between the time this introduction is

Introduction xxiii

written and the time this book is published. Because of the increasing cost of health care in general, and of mental health care delivery in specific, cost containment and cost-effectiveness have become paramount issues. Medicine is more and more regarded as an industry that offers a product, with the expectation that the whole enterprise will be made more efficient by competition, cost incentives, and the potential for profit. Increasingly, the societal goal is that acceptable health care be offered at the best price, rather than the best possible medical care be given with cost as a secondary concern. However, definitions of what is "acceptable" are subject to wide disagreement.

The past years have seen continuing and increasing movement toward managed care delivery of various sorts, although the degree to which health maintenance organizations (HMOs) and insurance systems that include care management have taken hold varies by geographic region. Currently, there may even be a leveling off or backlash against systems in which clinical care is "micro-managed" by managers remote from the clinical setting. There is a move toward management by "capitation," a system by which a group of providers assume the medical care of a panel of subscribers for a fixed per capita annual amount, with the possibility of profit, but also the risk of losses. The effects of this are not yet known.

In contemplating current health care—with increasing costs, increasing regulation (e.g., mandated ceilings on Medicare fees), aggressive competition between insurance providers (an estimated $4–$5 billion spent on health care marketing per year[*]), and the development of a three-tier care system (in which many millions have no access to health care)—growing numbers of health economists, politicians, professional medical organizations, and despite [the] failure of health reform in 1994, others predict some form of universal health insurance in the not too distant future. There is even talk about rationing health care. Regardless of which direction health care reform takes, in view of continuing increases in medical costs, it is likely that any system adopted will involve care management rather than direct and unlimited fee-for-service practice.

---

[*]David Himmelstein, M.D., personal communication, October 1994.

Within the uncertainties about health care delivery, there is even more uncertainty about psychiatric care, the stepchild of medical care, for which, under most plans and systems, coverage is more limited than for other medical care. One positive note is that some states are introducing "insurance parity" (i.e., equal coverage) for nonpsychiatric illnesses and severe or "biologically based" mental illnesses.

Contributing to the uncertainty for psychiatrists is the increase in numbers and in competition from other mental health professionals who are licensed to practice their professions independently in most states and to collect payment from third parties, and who are frequently sought because of their lower rates. In some states, psychologists are gaining—and certainly seeking—admitting privileges to hospitals; in addition, both psychologists and mental health nurses are seeking and obtaining prescribing privileges.

Choosing a Career Path in Psychiatry

A third time line is that of a career path. This book deals with training and career development in the various specialties and practice settings. In making plans, one has to consider length of training; whether training is full-time, as in a fellowship (e.g., child training, psychopharmacology), or is accomplished over some time concurrently with other professional activities (e.g., psychoanalytic training, group therapy training); how long it will take to establish oneself in a particular location, practice, or specialty; and whether one plans to follow one field of practice (e.g., emergency psychiatry, inpatient psychiatry) with another (e.g., private practice). Academic or administrative careers have a certain progression that generally depends on choices made early in one's career.

Personal Considerations

Finally, there is also a family time line. For many men and women, the years spent in training and early career development coincide with those spent establishing families, with the latter endeavor obviously requiring much energy and time. For women in particular, there is a need to deal with a biological time line. Even with new options and the viability of various lifestyles, most women physicians wish to marry or to bear children—or to do both. Despite an extension of the years during which women can now safely have children, for the majority, childbearing years coincide with the training and early posttraining years. Tension and conflict are virtually inevitable between "career grooming" and "family grooming" wishes and needs. Few women manage without conflict and without making some sacrifices in one or both areas. Several studies have shown that women psychiatrists perceive their main conflict to be between the demands of family and career. Often they postpone having children until after completion of training and then work fewer hours (approximately 20% fewer) than their male counterparts.

It is interesting, however, that even women without children tend to work fewer hours than men. Lifestyle and pursuit of other interests are more important to women, although recent data show that men, too, are becoming more concerned about lifestyle and family time.

To some extent, all chapters cover the history of their specialties or settings; the training offered or required for practice in them; organizations offering information, education, or support; and some of the special rewards as well as the problems associated with each specialty. Unbidden, all authors underscore the need for good basic clinical training and experience for practice in their specialty, and all delineate research opportunities in their fields. The specific ethical and legal tensions and potential problems within each type of practice also appear through almost all chapters and clearly warrant close attention by their practitioners.

Reference

Reiser MR: Are psychiatric educators "losing the mind"? Am J Psychiatry 145:148–153, 1988

For Further Reading

American Medical Association, Council on Long-Range Planning and Development: The future of psychiatry. JAMA 264:2542–2548, 1990

Persad E, Cameron P: Psychiatric training and the trainees: is there a fit? Can J Psychiatry 31:727–730, 1986

Schwartz RS: The double life of a psychiatrist: role changes between hospital and office. Psychiatry 50:83–87, 1987

Section I:
Research and Frontiers in Psychiatry

CHAPTER ONE

Psychiatric Research

Harold Alan Pincus, M.D.

Never before have there been so many opportunities for psychiatric research to advance psychiatrists' scientific knowledge base, nor has the potential for research to influence the clinical practice of psychiatry and care of the mentally ill ever been greater; and never before has public and political support of psychiatric research been so great. Yet, despite these opportunities, the prospect of research seems daunting and unobtainable for young physicians entering psychiatry. My purpose in this chapter is to demystify a research career, briefly describe some opportunities in the field, describe various elements that enter into becoming a psychiatric researcher, and, finally, answer specific questions about how to choose and use a research training program.

Perhaps no other field in biomedical research offers such tremendous opportunities as psychiatric research and neuroscience (Pincus et al. 1989). New techniques for neuroimaging and assessing brain activity and for understanding the processes of inter- and intracellular communication in the brain provide powerful methods for examining how the brain functions in health and disease. Advances in molecular biology, genetics, immunology, clinical and basic pharmacology, information systems, and other fields have relevance to psychiatry and enlarge psychiatrists' capacity to illuminate the mysteries of mental illness.

There has also been tremendous growth in the behavioral sciences related to psychiatry. The development of more reliable, specific, and valid methods for assessing behaviors, making diagnoses, conducting epidemiological studies, and assessing the outcome of psychotherapy provides psychiatrists with the ability to more carefully study the complex interactions between behavior and biology and to examine developmental pathways of psychiatric illness. Relatively new areas of research—mental health services research, for example—have grown tremendously and increased in influence. Assessment of outcomes of health care interventions in "the real world" has received a great deal of attention by health care policy makers (Roper 1988) to better define cost-effective care.

Opportunities for young investigators lie in areas of psychiatric research that have been insufficiently mined in the past, vast areas where truly significant contributions can be made, notably in child psychiatry research (Institute of Medicine 1989) and in alcohol and drug abuse research (Institute of Medicine 1987).

Public and political support is expanding as well. During the 1970s, research in mental health and psychiatry was often seen as unfocused, vague, and "soft," with research funding not keeping pace with inflation and in fact dropping in actual dollars. Political support for federal research funding dropped as it was not seen as fully relevant to patients with mental illnesses (Freedman 1985). In the late 1970s and early 1980s, however, respect for psychiatric research began to grow relative to the exciting opportunities described above and the increasing focus of research on those severe mental disorders that represented tremendous costs to patients, their families, and society as a whole. Organized citizens' groups representing psychiatric patients grew in size and potency, and placed research advocacy as a major focus on their agenda. Finally, the psychiatric research community became more organized and forceful in obtaining support for research on mental and addictive disorders.

In 1984, the Institute of Medicine issued a report documenting both past difficulties and growing opportunities in research on mental and addictive disorders. Since then, there has been an enormous turnaround in this area, manifested by 1) concrete changes in the level of support by both House and Senate appropriations committees responsible for funding research on mental and addictive disorders, and 2) a large expansion in the extramural research budgets of the National Institute of Mental Health (NIMH), National Institute on Drug Abuse, and National Institute on Alcohol Abuse and Alcoholism. There is also an increasing focus of this research funding on disorders that affect psychiatric patients, with significant growth in the proportion of funds going to departments of psychiatry. Currently, 51% of

NIMH research funds go to departments of psychiatry. Psychiatrists now represent approximately 34% of the principal investigators on NIMH grants, a proportion approximately equal to that of psychologists (during the 1970s, psychologists outnumbered psychiatrists as principal investigators on NIMH grants by a 2-to-1 ratio) (National Institute of Mental Health 1989).

Although the future looks bright for psychiatric research, obtaining research funding remains a highly competitive process requiring in-depth training and preparation. At the same time, psychiatric research represents an increasingly attractive career option. When compared with the current realities of clinical practice, there is a lessening difference in salary levels and "hassle" levels between research and clinical practice. Most clinical psychiatric investigators work in academic settings—usually in major medical centers; however, there are also opportunities in industry and in various independent or government-established research institutes. Other opportunities exist for psychiatrists to become involved in research administration, which may combine the actual conduct of research with administering federal, industry, or foundation research programs. In general, a career in research provides unusual flexibility, independence, and collegial interaction and the capacity to work on fascinating intellectual questions. Furthermore, young people entering psychiatric research will find themselves truly valued.

Attributes of the Psychiatric Clinician-Researcher[1]

How can the special characteristics of clinician-researchers be described in concrete terms for psychiatric residents or medical students gaining confidence in clinical skills and eager to pursue a research career? Burke et al. (1986) described five aspects of the professional role of psychiatric investigators:

---

[1]This section is adapted from Burke JD Jr, Pincus HA, Pardes H: "The Clinician-Researcher in Psychiatry." *Am J Psychiatry* 143:968–975, 1986.

1. A core clinical identity
2. An intellectual orientation toward science in order to investigate patterns of phenomena that elucidate facts of nature as well as individual characteristics
3. Technical skills to ask questions about the facts of nature rigorously and objectively
4. Management skills to organize such systematic inquiry in the clinic or laboratory
5. The values and motives of scientific medicine to make scholarly advances that will promote the prevention and healing enterprise

Core clinical identity. In the past, psychiatry, like other branches of medicine, has experienced a split between the two value systems of clinical practice and scientific research, between the images of soft-headed humanists and biological technocrats. Such a split implies two separate lines of development, with an inevitable tension between the two. It is important to view the psychiatric researcher as a clinician first, who learns to become a scientific investigator in addition to being a clinician. With this perspective, clinical thinking is no longer at odds with scientific inquiry; rather, patient care provides the basic underpinning to clinical research and vice versa.

Carroll (1984) argued that investigations of biological mechanisms in patients need to be conducted with a sophisticated sense of the nature of clinical phenomena. Simply applying the criteria listed in DSM-III (American Psychiatric Association 1980) as definitive guides to classification does not provide the strongest base for crucial questions, such as how to subtype heterogeneous conditions like schizophrenia and major depression. Clinical experience stands at the center of efforts to design, monitor, and interpret studies on treatment methods and their efficacy (Levine 1979) and to develop meaningful assessment techniques for measuring course and outcome (Waskow and Parloff 1974).

Major drawbacks, however, could derive from a clinician's continuing focus on individual patients rather than on larger groups of patients. Thinking in terms of anecdotal evidence may limit a psychiatric researcher's ability to abstract carefully from systematic inquiry on a targeted problem, or to balance empathy and intuition with rigorous objectivity and observation. Shifts between the individual and the "sample" may be difficult at times, but can be readily managed.

Consideration of the individual from a clinician's standpoint may be an advantage in dealing with issues such as informed calculations of risks and benefits to research subjects. Well-trained clinician-researchers seem best suited to manage the special problems of clinical studies, such as balancing clinical care with research protocols and defining appropriate control groups.

Intellectual orientation. Narrow-minded fascination with technical skills and statistical knowledge of research can produce "expert" investigators who are isolated from clinical or scientific reality. Research trainees must have powerful curiosity and creative energy to deal with scientific problems that are always challenging and often frustrating. Formal training entails learning a disciplined approach to scientific questions, developing intellectual strategies, and addressing problems that warrant study. Learning which questions to ask and how to ask them is much more important than mastering technical skills. Without a sense of the field and how to advance it, research effort can be wasted on meaningless correlations of complex data. In a time of high competition for research funding, not all "good" research is considered good enough to deserve support, necessitating the development of a coherent intellectual framework for approaching an area of research and developing strategies to answer the essential questions.

Technical skills. Beyond a general knowledge of research design and a workable knowledge of statistics, success can depend on mastery of particular techniques, whether biological assays or standardized diagnostic interviews. The problem for eager trainees is that often these technical skills seem to be all that is necessary, although they are only the tip of the training iceberg. An even greater danger is that commitment to just a few particular techniques can limit a scientist's vision and insidiously restrict his or her capacity to answer questions that have been identified.

Management skills. Research grant applications need more than a strong design in an important area. Peer reviewers are always concerned with whether a team of investigators can accomplish the work that seems so good on paper. Formulating a question with the proper integration of clinical perspective, sound intellectual strategy, and requisite technical skills is just the beginning. With the increased complexity of research projects and the need for a variety of skills on a research team, managing even a small study has become "big business." The principal investigator of any grant needs to be a successful manager of a series of interrelated tasks, a variety of professional and support personnel, and various institutional requirements set by the local institution and by government. Professionals who manage other enterprises receive training in schools of business or public administration. In science, the most successful investigators must also be able to exercise a high level of administrative skill, but typically without the benefit of formal training in these areas.

Consider the press of duties on a researcher who is a principal investigator: besides feverish efforts to complete applications and cope with site visits, there is a daily struggle to balance competing pressures of teaching, clinical responsibilities, administrative duties, and the conduct of ongoing research projects. Always in the background is the collection of unpublished results, which represents personal frustration as well as a waste of previously committed resources. There is a temptation to let the urgent replace the important, to let short-term demands take precedence over long-term responsibilities. In large and successful research enterprises, there is the danger of senior investigators losing contact with day-to-day operations, becoming little more than "absentee owners."

Successful management is more than administrative efficiency. With a variety of people involved, and often with the least-trained personnel responsible for day-to-day routines of dealing with subjects and even collecting important data, it is important for researchers to exercise the same executive leadership that Levinson and Klerman (1967) examined in relation to mental health service organizations. A capacity to motivate people and to sustain their enthusiasm and commitment is a major element of such leadership. Clinician-researchers must also interact at other administrative levels in the internal academic environment and with public and political representatives in order to communicate the importance of their work (Landau 1980).

Values and motives. It is essential for clinician-researchers to understand their own values and motives and to have a sense of what accomplishments are possible over the course of a career. Without a commitment to the work itself and to the ultimate goal of advancing the science of medicine, the values of an investigator facing these pressures may become distorted. In dramatic examples from general medicine, cases of outright fraud have been found in prestigious universities and multicenter studies (Broad 1982). Psychiatry has not been spared prominent examples of these tragic cases (American Psychiatric Association 1989).

Other problems are less dramatic but almost equally damaging to the long-term health of clinical research. Pressure to publish results dominates researchers in the effort to sustain promotions, create the image of a successful enterprise, justify continued funding, and support the next grant application. Young clinicians eager to make a name for themselves quickly need to learn the value of exercising restraint, carefully preparing data, and offering meaningful interpretations rather than rushing to get results into print.

Just as the values of science can be distorted by inadequate understanding and commitment to them, so can the clinical values that stand at the core of research. Investigators and their human subjects committees are expected to address whether potential benefits of a study outweigh its costs and whether informed consent has been freely given. Difficult questions often arise in monitoring clinical trials: for example, whether a protocol should be terminated before its anticipated completion if adverse effects become clear or a definite treatment advantage is demonstrated. The ability to consider such questions, which are likely to increase in the future, requires researchers to have thoughtful and balanced clinical perspectives and explicit ethical frameworks.

Becoming a Psychiatrist-Researcher

Choosing and Using a Research Training Program

In-depth scientific training is essential for all research, and psychiatry is no exception. In their recent study of full-time faculty in departments of internal medicine, Levey et al. (1988) indicated that those faculty members who were most successful in a research career (as measured by grants, publications, etc.) were those who had had at least 2 years of formal training and 3 additional years of protected support as they developed their research careers. Unfortunately, in psychiatry there has been a naïveté about the necessity of formalized research training (Haviland et al. 1987). Furthermore, unlike in other medical specialties, many teaching psychiatrists lack research training experience (e.g., potential mentors, ongoing participation in research). To achieve the capacity to function in the roles outlined earlier, future psychiatrist-researchers must be willing to train further in research.

Thus, formalized research training is a necessity for a successful career as a clinical investigator, though the notion that a Ph.D. degree is necessary to do good research is incorrect and unfortunate.

A number of programs varying in size and support exist to train psychiatrists as clinician-investigators. They share many common features such as concentrated involvement in research for at least 2 years, ongoing supervision by an experienced research mentor, and the presence of an active laboratory with sufficient resources and support. In examining research training programs, young people need to consider four principal questions to aid them in evaluating the utility and fit of particular programs:

1. By whom will I be trained (i.e., who will be available as possible mentors and what roles might the mentors assume)?
2. Where will that training take place (i.e., what are the institution's values and resources)?
3. With whom will I train (i.e., what will be the nature of collegial relations)?
4. How will the training take place (i.e., what will be the nature of the training itself)?

Role of the mentor. A program for research training cannot be easily reduced to a standard curriculum. What is needed is the consistent, intense, and close observation and interaction with a senior person who can provide guidance, advice, and substantive direction. In *The Odyssey,* Homer gave the name *Mentos* (meaning steadfast and enduring) to the friend whom Odysseus entrusted with the guidance and education of his son, Telemachus. Levinson et al. (1978) described the essential role of a mentoring relationship in the formative years of a young professional career:

> The mentor relationship is one of the most complex and developmentally important a man can have in early adulthood.... He [the mentor] may act as a teacher, ... sponsor, ... host and guide, [and] ... exemplar, ... [and] he may provide counsel and moral support.... The mentor has another function, and this is developmentally the most crucial one: to support and facilitate the realization of the Dream. The true mentor, in the meaning intended here, serves as an analogue in adulthood of the "good enough" parent for the child. (pp. 97–99).

Anecdotal stories abound regarding the importance of mentor relationships in the career paths of eminent people in all domains. In fast-moving, highly competitive fields such as scientific research, the mentor's role can be particularly significant. The problem facing young people is how to find a mentor. In general, it requires a considerable amount of effort, research, and luck. It is important that potential researchers read the literature with an eye toward identifying authors whom they particularly admire or find important, talk to people both at their home institution and at scientific meetings, and find out more about the mentoring style of senior people in programs they might be considering. A future researcher's own past relationships with teachers and advisers can help him or her discover what kind of relationship may work best.

Institutional values and resources. Personal and family issues and interests should be important in considering where one might undertake research training. From a professional perspective, however, there are three sets of questions to consider:

1. Does the institution have the necessary resources? Is there stability in the department in terms of a sufficient number of staff, facilities, and equipment? Is there sufficient diversification of funding, or an overdependence on a single source of support? In considering resources, a trainee should not simply focus on the presence of one or two pieces of high-technology equipment. Are the day-to-day

resources necessary to conduct research in the selected area sufficiently available? One should not have to rely on working out of "the kitchen sink."
2. What is the relationship between the psychiatry department and other departments at the institution? Are there strong collaborative research connections? Can resources of related departments be used to augment those of the psychiatry department?
3. Probably most important, are science and scientists highly valued in the department? Is there a tradition of excellence at the institution?

Nature of collegial relationships. Although there is evidence that programs with a large critical mass of faculty and trainees are most successful in producing researchers, many great scientists have also come from smaller institutions. One must consider one's own preferences in terms of "big fish/little pond versus little fish/big pond" issues. Many smaller programs that lack a sufficient critical mass within the department of psychiatry gain it by linking with other departments to maintain an extensive interdisciplinary research training program. Of course, research trainees are always part of a much larger community, connected in many ways through annual meetings, participation in various scientific organizations, and the scientific literature. Nevertheless, a basic factor is whether one respects and likes the colleagues with whom one will be trained. What was true from kindergarten through residency remains true for research training: much of what is learned is learned from peers.

Nature of the training itself. Two principal approaches to training have evolved. In the *Ph.D. model,* emphasis is on a defined curriculum that may lead to a formal degree, whereas the *apprenticeship model* emphasizes more experiential aspects of working collaboratively on a project with peers and mentors. Most programs are, in practice, combinations of these two approaches, although some are oriented more one way than the other. Again, individuals must appraise their own preferences in this regard, keeping balance in mind. Whereas it is essential that a potential trainee focus on technical aspects and understanding design, methodology, and statistics, he or she must also spend sufficient time with mentors and other colleagues and have time to develop an independent line of study. Anticipation of and preparation for life following the formal research training program are essential as well. Programs should address issues related to transition to an independent research career and incorporate practical aspects of linking with federal and other potential funding agencies, the mechanics of applying for research funding, and issues of practical management and administration of research projects.

Understanding Research Training From a Developmental Perspective

Research training is a developmental process beginning prior to and ending after the completion of any formal training program. During medical school or residency, exposure to an intensive research experience can offer an opportunity to assess talent and interest in a research career. Physicians can be provided with an uninterrupted period of basic research training and graduation to clinical training (Choppin 1989). Junior faculty need to be protected from excessive clinical duties to allow them to establish research programs and compete for grants.

The Role of the American Psychiatric Association

In 1985, the Office of Research was established at the American Psychiatric Association (APA) with the express purpose of taking a leadership role for the association in advancing science policy issues for psychiatry, systematizing and overseeing APA scientific assessment programs, and conducting and coordinating research at the APA. From the outset, issues in research training and the development of medical students and residents into future psychiatrist-investigators have been the highest priorities in the office. The office maintains close linkage with other components of the APA involved with residents and medical students and training issues in general, as well as with other organizations within and outside of psychiatry (e.g., American Association of Chairmen of Departments of Psychiatry, Association of American Medical Colleges, American College of Neuropsychopharmacology). *Psychiatric Research Report,* a quarterly newsletter, is published by the office and contains information about major science policy issues as well as a collection of research training and research funding opportunities for psychiatrists. A column specifically devoted to residents interested in research is in each issue. Anyone interested in a career in psychiatric research can receive *Psychiatric Research Report* free of charge.

With the support of the Van Ameringen Foundation, the APA has established a Psychiatric Research Resource Center to enhance the successful development of an enlarged cadre of psychiatrist-researchers. The center maintains a series of databases regarding research training opportunities and programs of funding and support for psychiatric research and can provide advice and linkage with other advisers and mentors for those considering psychiatric research careers.

In addition, the APA has established an extensive NIMH-funded program to attract minorities into careers in psychiatric research and to provide support (including funding for stipends, travel, tuition, and other expenses) for training experiences for medical students, residents, and postresidency fellows in major research-intensive departments of psychiatry.[2]

References

American Psychiatric Association: Diagnostic and Statistical Manual of Mental Disorders, 3rd Edition. Washington, DC, American Psychiatric Association, 1980

American Psychiatric Association, Office of Research: Dealing with scientific misconduct. Psychiatric Research Report 4:7, 1989

Broad WJ: Harvard delays in reporting fraud. Science 215:478–482, 1982

Burke JD, Pincus HA, Pardes H: The clinician-researcher in psychiatry. Am J Psychiatry 143:968–975, 1986

---

[2] For further information on these programs, for general advice and suggestions on research career opportunities, or to be placed on the mailing list for *Psychiatric Research Report,* contact the APA Office of Research, 1400 K Street, N.W., Washington, DC 20005.

Carroll BJ: Problems with diagnostic criteria for depression. J Clin Psychiatry 45:14–18, 1984

Choppin PW: Howard Hughes Medical Institute: training the next generation of medical scientists. Acad Med 64:382–383, 1989

Freedman DX: Research funds are down—take heart! Arch Surg 42:518–522, 1985

Haviland M, Pincus HA, Dial T: Career, research involvement and research fellowship plans of potential psychiatrists. Arch Gen Psychiatry 44:493–496, 1987

Institute of Medicine: Research on mental illness and addictive disorders: progress and prospects. Washington, DC, National Academy Press, 1984

Institute of Medicine: Causes and consequences of alcohol problems: an agenda for research. Washington, DC, National Academy Press, 1987

Institute of Medicine: Children and adolescents with mental, behavioral and developmental disorders: mobilizing a national initiative. Washington, DC, National Academy Press, 1989

Landau RL: Clinical research: elements for a prognosis. Perspect Biol Med 23:53–58, 1980

Levey G, Sherman C, Gentile N, et al: Postdoctoral research training of full-time faculty in academic departments of medicine. Ann Intern Med 109:414–418, 1988

Levine J (ed): Coordinating clinical trials in psychopharmacology: planning, documentation and analysis (DHEW Publ No ADM-79-803). Washington, DC, U.S. Government Printing Office, 1979

Levinson DJ, Klerman GL: The clinician-executive: some problematic issues for the psychiatrist in mental health organizations. Psychiatry 30:3–15, 1967

Levinson DJ, Darrow CN, Klein EB, et al: The Seasons of a Man's Life. New York, Knopf, 1978

National Institute of Mental Health: Research Information Source Book. Rockville, MD, National Institute of Mental Health, 1989

Pincus HA, Goodwin F, Barchas J, et al: The future of the science of psychiatry, in Future Directions for Psychiatry. Edited by Talbott J. Washington, DC, American Psychiatric Press, 1989, pp 75–106

Roper WL: Perspectives on physician-payment reform: the resource-based relative-value scale in context (editorial). N Engl J Med 319:865–867, 1988

Waskow IE, Parloff MB (eds): Psychotherapy change measures (DHEW Publ No ADM-74-120). Washington, DC, U.S. Government Printing Office, 1974

CHAPTER TWO

Zen and the Art of Biological Psychiatry Research

John M. Morihisa, M.D.

In deciding to pursue a career in biological psychiatry, it is useful to consider a variety of potential approaches and to have a knowledge of the obstacles, rewards, and sacrifices inherent in this career choice. This chapter, unlike Chapter 1, is subjective in that in it I pursue a case study approach to discussing careers in biological psychiatry research. This is, of course, just the opposite of the usual approach taken in this field, but perhaps as such it can offer a different point of view. My approach can, therefore, claim no statistical or generic validity but can only suggest a somewhat anthropological justification of meaning, as associated with participant observation. The reader is, therefore, warned to sample with care, with discrimination, and with a molecule of salt.

First, I consider some basic assumptions about education and offer a number of recommendations concerning this career path. Taken up within the context of these assumptions are basic training in the appropriate scientific disciplines, the range of one's educational experience, and the particular research arenas and experiences that might be usefully considered; all of this is presented, however, with the caveat that the paths to a successful career in biological psychiatry research are extremely variable, characterized at times by an innovative creativity.

Basic Training Assumptions

There is no question that a classical background in mathematics and biochemistry in undergraduate training with an additional course of study leading to a Ph.D. in molecular biology greatly enhance the ability of a physician trained in psychiatry to pursue some of the most interesting and challenging aspects of biological psychiatry research. However, this training carries no guarantee of a successful research career; likewise, neither is the pursuit of biological research in midcareer doomed without this background. Each situation merely defines the specific conditions that will pertain as one assesses career opportunities, research strategies, realistic goals, and the time frame for the achievement of those goals.

Regardless of when one decides to pursue biological research in psychiatry, the value of specific biological training cannot be overemphasized. Technological aspects of biological research have reached very complex proportions and are evolving at a logarithmic growth rate. The field is changing daily and techniques are being modified and enhanced constantly. Thus, specific, structured training in the biological approaches of interest is of the utmost importance.

In biological psychiatry research, it is valuable to receive training specifically in one's area of interest, although training in the basic scientific approach and the broad spectrum of theories that make up the research field is also needed. It is, however, absolutely essential to obtain specific training using the exact technique that will be applied in a particular research approach (e.g., positron emission tomography, histofluorescence microscopy, restriction fragment length polymorphisms). Without this essential training, researchers can inadvertently introduce numerous confounds, waste efforts, overlook basic methodological flaws, and apply inadequate bases for the development and refinement of the relevant theoretical framework. Indeed, without extensive hands-on experience in the specific area of biological research, one would be handicapped in much the same way as a clinician who attempted to master psychotherapy without seeing patients. During my residency training, my peers and I were often admonished that it takes at least 10 years of hard work and extensive clinical experience to produce a good psychotherapist. A similar time frame is important to the learning process of biological research, because learning experiences are continuing and evolving educational processes in which progress can be viewed over decades rather than months.

Personal Experience

At the Bronx High School of Science, my major interests were in mathematics and physics; I strongly considered a career in plasma physics in order to pursue the promise of cheap and environmentally clean fusion energy. However, in my senior year, I read some of the work of Sigmund Freud and vowed then to pursue the field of psychiatry, although my grasp of what actually constituted this field was limited. In applying to colleges, I clearly indicated that I was going to become a psychiatrist and was repeatedly counseled that this would destroy my chances of being accepted anywhere.

During a masterfully taught, fundamentally important Harvard College first-year seminar on the mind-body relationship, I learned that with the rapid advances in the neurosciences and psychopharmacology, medical training would be very valuable in the study of human behavior. As a medical student at the Mount Sinai School of Medicine, I had an opportunity to conduct basic science research under the mentorship of a pharmacology professor with an M.D. and a Ph.D. who had a brilliant grasp of research strategy and the establishment of research paradigms. Through allocation of most of my elective, vacation, and weekend time, and supported by summer research grants from the psychiatry and neurology departments, I was able to pursue basic science research in the dopamine system. Support from the psychiatry department and mentorship by the department chair were instrumental in refining my interests in the brain and behavior, both into a focus on psychiatry as a specialty and into the pursuit of basic science research on the brain.

After many months of careful investigation into the dopamine system, I could find absolutely no evidence of the phenomenon that I was trying to prove. At this crucial moment, my pharmacology research project mentor pointed out that, although I had failed to demonstrate what I had set out to do, these findings suggested something else of interest that could be pursued experimentally. At the time, I was struck by several fundamental points. First, I was appalled at my failure to perceive the basic scientific logic of this observation; but, at the same time, I perceived something special about science concerning the nature and potential value of carefully arrived at negative findings and findings that are opposite from what is expected. Secondly, it became apparent that experience and knowledge exert a powerful influence over conceptualization of research designs and interpretation of data. Finally, perhaps illogically, the opposite corollary seemed probable—that years of scientific investigation could lead to negative findings that go nowhere or only to work with ambiguous or uninterpretable meanings or no apparent application. Thus, the seductive dangers and potential delights of research were first introduced to me.

The results of these experiments were published in the journals *Nature* and *Brain Research* and gave me the confidence to make a very important decision concerning my residency at the Massachusetts Mental Health Center, where my first mentor was now the residency training director. My choice was to concentrate on developing expertise in clinical skills of psychiatry and to allocate my elective time to clinical areas rather than to research. In my final year, I elected not to pursue a research project but applied for a chief residency to give me important clinical administrative skills derived in large part from a seminar on administration given for chief residents by the center director. During my year as chief resident, I had the added advantage of having an outstanding teacher as an attending on my unit.

In large part, my decision to focus on clinical aspects of training was also aided by my prior application and acceptance to the National Institute of Mental Health (NIMH) clinical associate program. Knowing that I would be able to devote myself to research at the NIMH, I felt that residency would afford me the best opportunity to acquire clinical skills. It must be noted that doing basic science research in medical school had given me the necessary information to make a decision early in residency on eventually pursuing research training at the NIMH.

I enjoyed extraordinary good fortune in terms of superb teachers, mentors, and role models, as well as wonderful institutional support at crucial points in my career path. Added to this were the unparalleled resources of the NIMH intramural research program, with a critical mass of peers as well as mentors who nurtured the learning and research process. Despite this extraordinary mix of great people, mighty institutions, luck, and good fortune, it is my perception that this process was the most difficult task I ever set for myself, the most frustrating endeavor imaginable, and perhaps one of the most challenging to try to plan. The greatest challenges have not been to the mind but to the spirit. Indeed, in any area of psychiatry, one experiences great excitement, great frustration, much satisfaction, and some confusion and uncertainty. Nevertheless, this is the path psychiatrists choose and one that is ultimately most worthy, because we strive in our different approaches to alleviate some of the terrible suffering of our patients and their families. Who would not expect this task to present challenges and frustrations? But it also has rewards and satisfactions that nourish our spirits as healers.

Spirit and Character

It has become increasingly clear to me that two of the most important factors in a successful career in biological psychiatry research are character and spirit. (I admit that this is a subjective impression, unamenable to scientific logic or statistical analysis.) The rewards and satisfactions inherent in this career pathway can perhaps be most succinctly characterized by exploiting a Zen Koan. The applause one hears for the best scientific research is all too often the sound of one hand clapping. The best work is done alone in the laboratory or in writing papers. Clarity of purpose and dedication to rigorous scientific discipline are largely internal and personal phenomena rather than those of public acclaim. Many of the best scientists never win fame or prestigious scientific awards. Few psychiatrists have won Nobel Prizes or Lasker Awards (though this may change with the many talented scientists now committed to the field). Research is often lonely work that demands as much from family life as from individual discipline, although the best scientists often fight fiercely to balance scientific work with personal life, for without the equilibrium and perspective offered by family and friends, the scientific spirit can lose its keen edge.

The most difficult and spiritually demanding decisions in science are often made alone in the laboratory and go unrewarded and unrecognized, for they represent only what is expected in good science. The achievements of the very best scientists usually represent only the placement of a small brick in the foundation of science, and the true value of work is sometimes not clear for many decades. Indeed, scientific theories are routinely reevaluated and sometimes discarded as false long after a renowned scientist has passed from this sphere.

Thus, the rewards of research are not in public acclaim nor in dramatically and permanently changing the course of science. Instead, it is the intensely personal reward of a job well done and the creative satisfaction of strengthening a scientific design that are the most enduring gifts of this work. Contributions are gratifying in the context of the general shifting of the scientific process to a more productive path that leads eventually to better diagnostic and treatment approaches. For the best scientists, these gratifying phenomena often remain in the mind's eye rather than in public recognition, and are most accurately represented by the solitary satisfaction gleaned from the applause of "one hand clapping."

How to attain such spirit and character is one of the challenges of this career path. The search for these qualities is greatly assisted by the guidance of scientific mentors who have the wisdom and dedication to impart the perspective and judgment so vital to this work. One's years in high school and college are not too soon to seek out mentors, and the opportunity to gain new mentors with each new institution one attends is often an unharvested potential at each graduation. The value of multiple mentors is inherent in the fact that each has different strengths and interests and a distinctly different role in the development of a career. No one mentor has the "truth"; instead, each has been given a piece or an aspect of it, as in the Japanese story *Roshomon,* in which an incident is related four separate times using the viewpoint of a different character for each version. The different viewpoints present conflicting but equally compelling aspects of the truth, and it is by gathering up the experience of all these myriad truths that one can best prepare for the challenge of a research career.

One of my mentors at the NIMH once said that one of his jobs was to fire up my excitement when I was discouraged with the excruciatingly slow research process and, alternatively, to provide perspective when preliminary research findings appeared to promise the discovery of profound scientific truths. Balance and equilibrium are vital, as research is usually a long-distance race lasting decades rather than a sprint lasting a few minutes. Another similarity with Olympic sports is that much of the gratification and honor derive from the opportunity to participate rather than from the counting of medals and the quickly fading glory of victory.

Summary

The prospective candidate in this career path should get specific and formal experience in research—as a fellow at NIMH, as a research fellow at a university, or as a graduate student. Joys and satisfaction must derive from the work itself rather than from some hoped-for reward at the end of a series of successful experiments or at the end of one's career. Tangible rewards of medals, honors, and publications often come to those who stay the course, but often long after the true race has been run. Indeed, these public victories quickly fade in comparison with the abiding strength of the gratification of scientific work well done and a research design thoughtfully crafted. It is these simple joys that nourish and sustain the true scientist over the long journey. Because it is the journey that is ultimately important rather than the final destination, it is these basic satisfactions that the prospective biological psychiatrist-researcher should search for in making career decisions. This search must begin and end in the spirit and character of the individual.

It is perhaps most succinct to suggest that a career is more similar in its nature to life than to science. There are unpredictable obstacles and delightful surprises but little apparent order inherent in the pursuit of a career in biological psychiatry research. Perhaps the most important quality in nurturing success is the strength to constantly reassess and review, then change one's mind and try a new and completely different tack.

Finally, although recent neuroscience research suggests that this basic ability might be intertwined in neuroanatomic structures as specific as the neural networks of the dorsolateral prefrontal cortex, it is as yet beyond our science to determine what subtle differences in brain function allowed an Einstein to overcome his initial difficulties in mathematics and then go on to shake the foundations of atomic physics and open a new arena of scientific endeavor. Indeed, something will be indefinably lost when this distinction may be made scientifically. For now it must be subsumed under the unscientific category of spirit.

CHAPTER THREE

Psychopharmacology

George W. Arana, M.D.
Laura Rames, M.D.

Psychopharmacology has become a major component in the general practice of psychiatry. It is essential that all psychiatrists become versed in managing psychiatric patients with psychotropic agents. The recent explosion in neurosciences research and neuropharmacology makes it imperative that all psychiatrists learn the indications and uses of pharmacotropics, especially as psychiatrists increasingly become regarded as leaders in the multidisciplinary mental health treatment team.

Careers in the areas of psychopharmacology span a wide spectrum of opportunities—from the laboratory bench and the study of molecular genetics, receptor kinetics, pharmacodynamics, pharmacokinetics, and so on, to the general practicing psychiatrist who chooses to concentrate on the treatment of psychiatric illness with pharmacotropics. Specialization in psychiatric pharmacology can range from a private practice with a specific interest or expertise (e.g., lithium, antidepressants) to a laboratory-oriented psychiatrist undertaking research as a molecular biologist investigating receptor subtyping.

History of Psychopharmacology

The field of psychopharmacology can be divided into early psychopharmacology and modern psychopharmacology. The advent of modern psychopharmacology came with the use of opiates and barbiturates for management of acute behavioral difficulties in patients; at this stage, psychopharmacology was a nonspecific art in which sedation was often the active component of behavioral control. The modern era of psychopharmacology emerged in the early 1950s with the development of chlorpromazine for psychotic illnesses, the beginning of the use of lithium carbonate for mania, and, in rapid succession, the development of tricyclic antidepressants, monoamine oxidase inhibitors, benzodiazepines, and a variety of antipsychotics and antidepressants similar to the medicines named above.

During the 1950s and 1960s, psychiatry was a strongly psychoanalytically oriented field in which the origins of pathological thoughts and behaviors were thought to be grounded in early life experience. Against this background, efforts were made to improve the study of the efficacy of psychopharmacological compounds. At that time, the outcome variables in the assessment of these agents were not part of "hard science" (i.e., there were no laboratory tests for assessing efficacy or specific, measurable biological entities). Placebo-controlled, blinded studies, in which patients are treated with the new active compound and investigators are blinded to the content of the medicines being administered, also mark the beginning of modern psychopharmacology. As antipsychotics, antidepressants, and lithium were more carefully studied—with the development of methods for analyzing blood levels with respect to clinical outcome and with increased sophistication in the clinical trials of these medicines—it became more and more apparent that specific compounds were able to ameliorate the major symptoms of acute and chronic syndromes quite predictably.

In the early 1960s, Dr. Julius Axelrod was awarded the Nobel Prize in biochemistry for his proposed model of synaptic transmission of nerve signals; his theory was revolutionary and had a profound impact on research in the neurosciences. What followed was a virtual explosion of biochemical brain research into the effects of psychotropic agents on brain chemistry and the testing of many hypotheses (e.g., dopamine hypothesis for schizophrenia, the adrenergic hypothesis for depression).

During the first 15 years when psychotropic compounds were being developed, many of the psychiatrists who studied them were learning laboratory methodology and biochemical principles in an informal way. Many of these psychiatrists had been trained as psychoanalysts and took an interest in psychiatric medications because of effects they saw with these compounds in specific clinical situations. After the 1960s, more trainees in psychiatry became interested in the indications for and efficacy of medications and began to specialize in the use and toxicities of these compounds (Coryell 1987; Garfinkel et al. 1979).

The 1970s and 1980s were further marked by increased sophistication in the development of the neurosciences, with a better understanding of the synaptic aspects of the action mechanism of drugs. Presently, psychopharmacology is entering into an exciting era in which techniques of molecular pharmacology are being applied to understand the effect of drugs on molecular systems and the parameters that are critical for predicting response to certain antipsychotics and antidepressants.

Opportunities in Psychopharmacology

As in most psychiatry, a pure practice in any of the following options is the exception rather than the rule; most psychopharmacologists practice in a situation involving some combination of these.

Full-time research. Although all fields of medicine demand excellent researchers, psychiatry and the neurosciences remain the "new frontier" of medical scientific study, with exciting advances every day. The creative, curious, patient, and dedicated physician is well suited for this work. Full-time research necessitates association with an academic facility or a pharmaceutical firm, both of which offer the advantages of continuing education, support services, and opportunities for shared participation in projects. A large referral base and a varied patient population are also advantageous. This does not necessarily require one to live in a large city, but cities often are the setting for these facilities. One frustrating aspect of research in an academic setting is that the patients referred to these tertiary care facilities often include a preponderance of atypical cases and/or patients who do not respond to available treatments. This skewed population of difficult-to-treat patients can present overwhelming challenges to the researcher. The gratification in discovery of improved treatment options, however, is the reward that makes treating this group worth the effort.

Full-time, hospital-based practice. Psychopharmacological expertise is in high demand in state hospitals and wards for the chronically mentally ill. The most severely ill patients are often the ones who experience the most profound improvements from psychotropic medications, thus providing the treating psychiatrist with a most gratifying experience. Sheer numbers of patients and a wide variety of pathology prevent this type of practice from becoming mundane. It is unfortunate that state facilities are often far removed from academic departments of psychiatry. To address this problem, some states have implemented academic psychopharmacological teaching programs for clinicians in their psychiatric facilities. Fully trained psychopharmacologists with teaching interests are in great demand in these settings (Green et al. 1989), and highly motivated, independent, and innovative individuals could thrive in this environment. However, because a psychopharmacologist practicing in such a setting might be isolated from an academic center, disciplined independent study, frequent seminar attendance, and planned interactions with other psychopharmacologists are required to maintain expertise in the field.

Private practice. Private practice allows the psychiatrist specially trained in medication management the unique opportunity to be a consultant to other psychiatrists as well as psychologists, social workers, or other mental health specialists. Of foremost importance is the education of colleagues, which can be a difficult undertaking requiring tact and empathy. Most medication failures are not attributable to improper medication but rather to underdosing or overdosing by practitioners, an insufficient course of time on medication, and poor compliance on the part of the patient. Everyone, even psychiatrists, would like a "quick fix" for difficult patients; the expert's best recommendation in these situations is often encouragement to continue the treatment already prescribed with minor adjustments.

Community-based practice. In this setting, the psychopharmacologist sees a mixture of inpatients and outpatients and mainly focuses on ways to use medications to allow patients to stay in the community. It is unfortunate that innovative treatment plans arrive in this setting slowly, but offer abundant opportunities for the specialist to rapidly incorporate improvements in existing treatments. Multidisciplinary treatment teams to follow patients' social and economic concerns (and even to make home visits, if necessary) are available in some cities. The well-trained psychopharmacologist can provide leadership or consultation to such teams for immeasurable benefits.

Training Requirements and Opportunities

Although presently no board certification exists for psychopharmacology as a subspecialty, there are many fellowships around the country offering positions in research and clinical specializations. Moreover, medical students planning to do a psychiatric residency with special interest in psychopharmacology would do well to search for programs using the following guidelines.

Quality of the department. Be it an advantage or disadvantage, most National Institute of Mental Health (NIMH) grant money is awarded to only a small number of psychiatry departments. About three-quarters of all grants are obtained by only about 10% of departments (Baldessarini 1990). As NIMH is the primary source for federally approved funding in psychiatry, this is an important consideration. Therefore, a measure of the competence of a given program to teach "cutting edge" psychopharmacology is the amount of extramural grant support it receives. This information can be obtained from the research faculty, and a well-funded program would be proud to provide this information.

Available faculty. Ideally, the program should offer exposure to faculty involved in "wet lab" research, which deals with the preclinical phase of psychotropic medication testing as well as neurotransmitters, genetics, animal research, and so on. Faculty should also be involved in clinical research of new medications and have a desire to supervise residents as either co-researchers of major projects or principal investigators of more limited studies.

Clinical experience. In the past, psychiatry has suffered from a division that produces two separate tracks in psychiatric training: the practitioner (clinician) and the scientist (researcher). This early over-specialization inhibits the development of both the objective, innovative clinician and the empathic, socially committed researcher. We agree with Burke et al.'s (1986) assumption that psychiatric researchers must be clinicians first who learn to become scientific investigators as well. Therefore, even if psychopharmacological research is one's ultimate avocation, quality clinical experience is an essential prerequisite.

Students of psychopharmacology should be exposed to well-supervised instruction from the beginning of their residency. We have found that the following model provides excellent training. When the resident is on the hospital inpatient wards, patient-resident-supervisor contact is essential early in training to help the student learn to separate idiosyncratic symptoms from specific symptoms of well-known syndromes (McHugh 1987). Although daily rounds with an attending physician allow adequate day-by-day evaluation of medications, an additional 90 minutes weekly of psychopharmacology case presentation is helpful. In this setting, patients with complicated medication management are interviewed by a psychopharmacology supervisor in front of residents and students, allowing ample time for teaching, questions, and discussion. As residents move to the outpatient clinic setting, this same close contact with a supervisor is recommended. Ideally, a 2- to 4-hour weekly clinic should be developed for those patients requiring medication management. Each supervisor should evaluate all patients in the clinic and be available for questions from and consultation to residents. This will allow a resident to obtain a "longitudinal view" of medication management not available in the acute hospital setting, as well as encourage the resident to develop independent thinking and decision-making skills.

Patient population. It is essential that trainees see a broad spectrum of patients—with a wide range of diagnoses, ages, and socioeconomic statuses—in order to receive a diverse learning experience. A training program should provide access not only to tertiary level patients so often referred to a university, but also to patients in Veterans Administration hospitals, state or county hospitals (Green et al. 1989), and possibly private hospitals, to incorporate all aspects of psychiatric pathology. In addition, because one-quarter to one-third of psychiatric patients have concomitant medical illnesses and are treated with many medications, exposure via consultation-liaison psychiatry is also recommended.

Additional considerations. Students of psychopharmacology should become scholars of their field early in training. In-depth literature searches in specific areas of interest as well as participation in journal clubs for literature discussion are optimal and are recommended not only for training but as lifelong activities, as continuing education is probably more crucial in psychopharmacology than in any other area of psychiatry. New medications are introduced frequently and specialists must keep abreast of innovative therapies.

When searching for a training program or fellowship, one should also inquire whether involvement in national or area meetings is encouraged. Not only does such involvement provide opportunities for presentation of research results or case studies, but it also enriches one's learning by allowing exposure to recent findings by researchers in other programs. Also, the experience of networking with others with similar interests is invaluable; multicenter collaboration in research, discovery of future employment options, and introduction to premier investigators in the field are but a few of the opportunities made possible by attending such meetings.

Economics of Psychopharmacology

Clinical aspects. It is quite clear that in an era of increased complexity of psychotropic drugs, a clinical practitioner who develops expertise in the use of these compounds would be valuable to any group practice or in any community. Generally speaking, psychopharmacology consultants in general practice charge fees in the same range as those of psychotherapists and psychoanalysts.

Research aspects. Psychiatrists going into clinical research of psychopharmacological compounds would be best served to train in a center where there are senior faculty undertaking this particular line of research. The economics of this work, of course, are variable and depend on the institution where that member was training; often the more senior faculty experts have large clinics where trainees can learn "at the bedside" and can also enhance salaries with private fees.

Laboratory research. The psychiatrist interested in specializing in laboratory-based psychopharmacology research would most likely need to be working in a research center at a university or in a pharmaceutical house. It is important to understand that much of the funding for preclinical psychopharmacology offers an income that is more modest than that of the practitioner or clinical psychopharmacologist.

Special Legal Considerations

Psychopharmacologists often are asked to consult on complicated issues (e.g., treatment of resistant affective, psychotic, and anxiety disorders) and thus often may have more complicated caseloads than the general practitioner in psychiatry. Because some psychotropic drugs have major toxicities with potentially lethal effects at high doses or in medically compromised individuals (e.g., cardiac problems with tricyclics, overdose potential with monoamine oxidase inhibitors and benzodiazepines, abuse potential of some compounds), psychopharmacologists must be cautious about recommendations, documentation, and the manner in which they explain the consultations and the patient's options. Increasingly, forensic psychiatrists and legal consultants recommend the use of informed consent for treatments with certain drugs, whereas 10 years ago this was not an issue. The psychopharmacologist-in-training needs to be aware of rapidly changing practice patterns and legal consequences in order to advise colleagues.

Specific Study Populations

It is critical that more individuals who enter the research field of psychopharmacology be aware of the special needs of specific population groups. In particular, there is now a growing area of psychopharmacology focusing on the toxicities of certain compounds, such as lithium and neuroleptics in Asian populations, including issues related to blood level of drug and optimal range (Blackwell 1977). It would be essential for similar research to be conducted in African-American, Hispanic, Native American, and other minority populations. In addition, little has been done in the field of psychopharmacology regarding the specific problems, efficacies, and toxicities of these drugs in women as compared with those in men.

Conclusion

Psychopharmacology is a rapidly growing subspecialty of psychiatry. Its large database is constantly changing, so that specific training starting in residency is essential for the individual planning to pursue this specialty. We recommend that anyone interested in psychopharmacology as a subspecialty take at least a 1-year (preferably a 2-year) postresidency fellowship in order to increase his or her exposure to a large variety of patients and to consolidate his or her knowledge base under supervised conditions.

References

Baldessarini RJ: The future of psychiatric research and academic psychiatry. McLean Hospital Journal 15:53–68, 1990
Blackwell B: Culture, morbidity, and the effects of drugs. Clin Pharmacol Ther 19:79–86, 1977
Burke JD, Pincus HA, Pardes H: The clinician-researcher in psychiatry. Am J Psychiatry 143:968–975, 1986
Coryell W: Shifts in attitudes among psychiatric residents: serial measures over 10 years. Am J Psychiatry 144:913–917, 1987
Garfinkel P, Cameron P, Kingstone E: Psychopharmacology education in psychiatry. Can J Psychiatry 24:644–651, 1979
Green A, Bennett M, Salzman C: An extramural training program in psychopharmacology: one model for a state system. Hosp Community Psychiatry 40:126–127, 1989
McHugh PR: William Osler and the new psychiatry. Ann Intern Med 107:918–924, 1987

CHAPTER FOUR

Sleep Disorders Medicine (Somnology)

Milton Kramer, M.D.

> Sleep, . . . balm of hurt minds. . . .
>
> Shakespeare, *Macbeth*

An interest in sleep is inevitable for psychiatrists because changes in sleep and disturbances of sleep are so frequent in the patients they see. Difficulties in falling asleep experienced by anxious patients and in staying asleep experienced by depressed patients are part of psychiatric clinical experience. Sleeplessness may herald the onset of an acute schizophrenic episode, and the beginning of undisturbed sleep signals the return to normalcy in delirious and manic patients. Furthermore, psychiatrists' interest in and understanding of the workings of the mind have been shaped by the insights of Freud, who built his model of the mind on the examination of his patients' dreams.

Development of Psychiatry's Interest in Sleep

The discovery of the biological basis for dreaming by Kleitman, Aserinsky, and Dement (Aserinsky and Kleitman 1953; Dement and Kleitman 1957) offered to fulfill the promise made by Hughlings Jackson, Jung, and Freud that if psychiatrists could understand the dream, "the sane man's psychosis" (Jung 1964), they might be on their way to understanding (and, consequently, curing) schizophrenia. Although that particular promise has not been realized, the identification of rapid eye movement (REM) sleep—a particular subpart of sleep—has contributed fundamentally to psychiatry's understanding of common entities such as depression and unusual ones such as narcolepsy. REM sleep is characterized by 1) visual dreaming as a common, if not inevitable, accompaniment; 2) recurrence at regular intervals across sleep, and probably across the entire 24-hour period; 3) a great deal of autonomic instability; and 4) a unique ontogenetic, phylogenetic, and developmental profile. The discovery of REM sleep has spurred a reexamination of the phenomenon of dreaming (Kramer 1990).

In the 1960s, as the mysteries of psychosis were being unraveled, psychiatrists were drawn to the fundamental observation of the recurrent periodic occurrence of REM sleep. A core group of these psychiatrists met for the first time at the University of Chicago in 1961 to share their observations about REM sleep. From that point, interest in the phenomenon of sleep has grown at an astounding rate, with the development of both research and clinical laboratories and through work by members of various disciplines (i.e., psychiatrists, neurologists, psychologists, physiologists, ethologists, and other neuroscientists).

In 1963, the second edition of Kleitman's book *Sleep and Wakefulness* was published; it contained over 4,000 references and summarized the then-current world literature on sleep. By the late 1960s, the sleep research community was publishing several thousand articles and books annually, thus indicating the explosion of new knowledge that observations about REM sleep created.

Up to the early 1970s, basic scientific information that had been learned about sleep was unsystematically applied to patients by research clinicians. In 1975, the Association of Sleep Disorders Centers (ASDC) was organized to establish standards for sleep disorders centers and to develop the application of knowledge of sleep to the diagnosis and treatment of sleep disorders. (The ASDC became the American Sleep Disorders Association [ASDA] in 1987.) The diagnosis and treatment of narcolepsy and of the then newly described condition of obstructive sleep apnea (Gastaut et al. 1966) became a focus of interest for sleep clinicians. A diagnostic nomenclature of sleep disorders was developed in 1979 and revised in 1990 (ASDA 1990). By 1992, there were more than 187 sleep disorders centers that were certified to adhere to standards developed by the ASDA.

Somnology and Psychiatry Today

The new knowledge that has been gained about sleep and sleep-related disorders makes it imperative that physicians be knowledgeable about sleep, be able to make an appropriate diagnosis, and be able to treat sleep disorders properly. With a 17% incidence of severe insomnia in the adult population, half of which is emotionally based (Mellinger et al. 1986), and with excessive daytime sleepiness affecting perhaps 3% of the adult population (Gallup poll—"Wake Up America," 1991), sleep disorders services are and will be needed in general and psychiatric hospitals as well as in academic departments of psychiatry. The clinical need is enormous, the opportunities are available, and specialty trained physicians are in great demand.

The major clinical-research challenge is in understanding the behavioral alterations occurring during sleep: sleepwalking, REM behavior disorders, somnological (nocturnal) epilepsy, dissociative states, and enuresis. The role of sleep in schizophrenia, circadian disorders of sleep (Foulkes 1985), and the application of light treatment to sleep disorders are other promising developments.

A reexamination of psychiatrists' understanding of the process of dreaming has been an inevitable concomitant of the discovery of the so-called biological substrate for dreaming—REM sleep. Efforts to examine the parallelism between the psychological and biological events occurring during REM sleep have not been particularly illuminating; dream reports have been recovered from all stages of sleep, undercutting the view of dreaming as only an REM stage phenomenon.

In keeping with the "new look" at mental phenomena that the cognitive revolution (Brunner 1990) has spurred, dreaming as a psychological process has begun to be the focus of research efforts. Much experimental work on dreaming was reexamined by Foulkes (1985) and Arkin et al. (1978) from a cognitive point of view. LaBerge (1985) explored the experience of awareness during dreaming, and lucid dreaming has become a topic of considerable interest. The current view of dreaming that has emerged is that dreams reflect as well as affect individuals' behavior. Cartwright's (1990) studies of dreams of divorced people showed that their dream content reflected the quality of their adaptation to being divorced. In individuals with a poor adaptation, manipulation of the dream experience facilitates improvement in the quality of their adaptation.

New theories of dreaming have been offered, and have been collected in a work edited by Moffitt et al. (1993), which is part of a series on dreams edited by Van de Castle. For example, Kramer (1993) stated that dreaming serves as a selective modulator of affective states, much like an emotional thermostat. New ideas about the meaning of dreams were described by Kramer and Roth in "Dream Translation" (1977) and by Delaney in *Living Your Dreams* (1979), the latter being an existentialist-Jungian approach to dream interpretation. Working with dreams in groups from an educational framework was described by Ullman and Zimmerman in their book *Working With Dreams* (1979).

Research is needed on the construction of dreams. What are the rules by which events (e.g., thoughts, feelings, memories) are selected and transformed to be included in dreams? Further, what principles then guide the combining of these elements into the dream experience? An approach to dreams that views dreaming as part of the narrative abilities of the dreamer, as States (1993) suggested ("the dreamer's personal fiction"), may offer the greatest promise of expanding our knowledge of dreams and the process of dreaming.

Working as a Somnologist

Psychiatrists specializing in sleep disorders can apply their knowledge of sleep to clinical practice by providing consultation to their psychiatric colleagues or to nonpsychiatric physicians in a consultation-liaison relationship, or by practicing with other sleep specialists in a multispecialty sleep disorders center. In the future, it is expected that clinical sleep disorders services will be developed in most, if not all, hospital settings and in many freestanding settings as well. In addition, home monitoring of sleep will certainly increase. Services will be provided to remote sites with the development of new, more portable monitoring techniques with automatic scoring.

The model for work I advocate and describe in this chapter is one of psychiatrists devoting a major portion of time to the subspecialty practice of somnology (sleep disorders medicine). Despite great clinical need, well-informed clinicians are not readily available.

The hospital-based center in which I practice is a complete service unit for the diagnosis and treatment of all sleep disorders. It has the capacity to study the sleep of eight patients per night. The center's medical director is a psychiatrist-somnologist and an accredited clinical polysomnographer who sees 175 new patients a year and evaluates 1,800 polysomnograms.[1] The center employs a manager, a receptionist, a clerk, a typist, seven polysomnographic technicians, and two part-time nurse clinical specialists who provide behavioral treatment for enuresis, insomnia, and nightmares.

As the director, my work includes evaluating new patients, reading and reviewing patients' polysomnographic records with staff, planning further diagnostic steps, and seeing patients for treatment and follow-up. There are administrative obligations, meetings, and hospital consultations. Time can be allotted to research and writing; to participating in educational activities for medical students, residents, colleagues, and even lay groups; to maintaining some general psychiatric outpatient practice; and to pursuing other professional interests.

The following is a description of a typical case I might see in the center:

> Mr. A, a 45-year-old truck driver, fell asleep while driving and crashed into a telephone pole. No one was hurt, but he had his driver's license suspended and was unable to work thereafter. When seen at a sleep disorders center, he was distraught and tearful.
>
> Mr. A had had diabetes since his teenage years, with continued hypoglycemic episodes. He had gained 20 pounds in the 2 years before the accident. His wife was unable to sleep in the same room with him because of his loud snoring, something over which they had arguments. In addition, he had become impotent.
>
> Mr. A went to the bathroom several times a night and fell back asleep easily. He was a restless sleeper and complained of discomfort in his legs; his frequent leg movements were another reason his wife gave for not sleeping with him. On physical examination, he was overweight at 5 feet 10 inches and 240 pounds. His upper airway showed considerable posterior tonsillar pillar webbing. His neurological examination was unremarkable.

---

[1] *Polysomnography* refers to the continuous and simultaneous monitoring and recording of various physiological parameters during sleep.

The differential diagnosis for Mr. A included obstructive sleep apnea, restless legs, nocturnal myoclonus, an interruption insomnia secondary to stress (depression), a seizure disorder, and diabetes with hypoglycemia. The patient was evaluated with 2 nights of polysomnography, a multiple sleep latency test (Kramer 1988, 1989), the Minnesota Multiphasic Personality Inventory (MMPI; Hathaway and McKinley 1970), lateral neck films recumbent, radiographic cephalometry, complete blood count, arterial blood gases, fasting blood sugar, thyroid panel, and electroencephalogram (EEG). The results showed 275 myoclonic jerks the first night and 320 the second, with an arousal index of 60%. There was no evidence of obstructive sleep apnea. Mr. A's REM latency was 70 minutes on one night and 120 minutes on another. He had 15 spontaneous arousals on his first night and 19 on his second. He fell asleep in 3 minutes the first night and in 7 minutes the second. The multiple sleep latency test showed a mean sleep onset time of 4.7 minutes, where 5 minutes or less is pathological sleepiness and 10 minutes or above is normal. The MMPI suggested a stable character disorder. His EEG was normal. The only other positive finding was an elevated morning blood sugar of 160.

Mr. A was found to have nocturnal myoclonus and was started on low doses of clonazepam (Klonopin) 0.5 mg, 1–4 tablets, 1 hour before bedtime. His sleepiness disappeared, and at 6-month follow-up his nocturnal myoclonus had been reduced to 50 myoclonic jerks, with an arousal index of 20% and a mean sleep onset time across five naps of 9 minutes. During the 6-month period, Mr. A's diabetes was stabilized under the care of his family physician, and he lost 22 pounds. He returned to work without difficulty. He and his wife were sleeping together, as his limb movements had become minimal and undisturbing. Mr. AA's snoring was a problem only occasionally. His impotence had not improved.

Satisfactions, Problems, and Frustrations in Somnology

The case of Mr. A captures a bit of the intellectual process engaged in by the somnologist. Taking a history, enumerating the possibilities, ordering proper examinations, establishing the correct diagnosis, testing the diagnosis with appropriate therapeutic intervention, and having a follow-up for confirmation provide a model for much of what is intellectually satisfying in clinical work in general and somnology in particular. A case like that of Mr. B's, which follows, illustrates the satisfactions of continued learning from one's own clinical experience.

Mr. B, a 51-year-old man, came to a sleep disorders center for treatment of narcolepsy. His sleep attacks and muscle weakness, which occurred when he became excited, had begun when he was in high school. He had been treated with amphetamines for sleepiness and with a tricyclic for his cataplexy. In the previous 10 years, his muscle weakness had increased; for the past 2 years, he had needed to stop even on brief walks or going up two flights of stairs because of pain in his legs.

The somnologist found the intensified cataplexy to be unusual and unlikely to account for Mr. B's increased fatigue on exertion. Following referral to a neurologist, Mr. B was diagnosed with McArdle's disease (Kramer and McGinnis 1986), an autosomal recessive disease in which there is an abnormal accumulation of glycogen in skeletal muscle because of the absence of the enzyme myophosphorylase *b*. This diagnosis was confirmed by muscle biopsy.

Entrance into somnology for a general psychiatrist represents an abrupt return to clinical medicine. The breadth of problems encountered ranges from illnesses such as primary or secondary insomnia to cardiorespiratory problems of obstructive apnea, sleep problems of infants and their mothers, bed-wetting problems of latency-age children, and nocturnal epilepsy, to the differential diagnosis of psychological versus organic impotence, and paroxysmal nocturnal dyspnea or gastroesophageal reflux in a patient awakening with chest pain.

The greatest satisfaction for the psychiatrist-somnologist results from the relatively definitive capacity for effective diagnosis and treatment using objective diagnostic tools. In a field such as psychiatry, which still seeks objective diagnostic tools, somnology offers a new and exciting contrast. To grow with a field still close to its beginnings is another obvious source of pleasure.

Major problems in somnology are associated with one of the field's major sources of satisfaction. The newness of the field, which offers the excitement of discovery, has as its concomitant an unevenness of acceptance by medical colleagues and third-party payers. Physicians who act as evaluators or consultants for plans involving managed care often are ill informed about sleep problems and inappropriately limit valuable diagnostic and therapeutic interventions by somnologists.

Education and Professional Organizations

Education

The major limitation in preparing for the practice of somnology is the highly variable nature of the training experience. As yet, no national body systematically evaluates and certifies training sites. However, excellent training is available in many sleep disorders centers, a listing of which is available from the ASDA.

Training in somnology must include diagnosis and treatment of an adequate number of patients of all ages and in all diagnostic categories in a full-service sleep disorders center, with adequate time for studying these patients. It should entail knowledge of all evaluation equipment currently in use. Somnologists must learn to score polysomnographic records for all current parameters (e.g., sleep stages and latencies, apneic and myoclonic episodes, changes in penile circumference and rigidity) (Rechtschaffen and Kales 1963). Familiarity with and involvement in collection of data in the laboratory are essential to adequate training in order for the trainee to appreciate the limitations of methodology.

Trainees must have time to study texts that give an overview of sleep disorders medicine (Kryger et al. 1989; Reite et al. 1990) as well as the research literature. The development, execution, and write-up of a clinical or basic science research project should be part of all somnology fellowships. Some time should be devoted to the administrative aspects of funding and staffing and to involvement in public and professional education. Training requires time. One month is not adequate; a year, properly utilized, probably is.

There is an examination for certification as a specialist in sleep medicine that requires some training experience and both basic science and clinical knowledge. Currently, this certifying board exists separately from the American Medical Association's Accreditation Council for Graduate Medical Education and includes nonphysicians with a doctoral equivalent. However, there has been some movement toward separating the board examination into one for physicians and one for nonphysicians. The increasing medicalization of somnology as a clinical practice is a welcome development.

Professional Organizations

There is one umbrella organization, the Association of Professional Sleep Societies (APSS), that brings together professionals as well as technical-level persons who are interested in the study of sleep. The

APSS is composed of three groups: the American Sleep Disorders Association (ASDA), currently with more than 230 fellows, which is for professionals—both physicians and nonphysicians—who are interested in the clinical application of knowledge about sleep; the Sleep Research Society (SRS), which is for professionals who are interested in and engaged in research about sleep; and the Association of Polysomnographic Technologists (APT), which is a technical group comprising nonprofessionals who do sleep recordings. The first two groups have overlapping membership. There are a number of publications related to the APSS: the official publication, the journal *Sleep,* a quarterly newsletter, and a newsletter published by the APT. The volume *Sleep Research* is published annually (Chase et al. 1972–1994) and encompasses the abstracts of the annual APSS meeting and an updated literature survey for the year.

APSS is affiliated with groups such as the European Sleep Research Society, the Japanese Sleep Research Society, and the Latin American Sleep Research Society. The APSS holds a meeting in the United States annually and an international meeting every 4 years. There also are regional sleep societies.

The widespread interest in dreaming as a psychological event led some 6 years ago to the development of the Association for the Study of Dreams. This 500-member group has both professional and lay members, holds an annual meeting, publishes a newsletter, and, as of 1991, has published a professional journal, *Dreaming*.

Economic Aspects of Somnology

The most frequent mode of practice for subspecialists in somnology is as medical director of a hospital-based sleep disorders center. The medical director's role may be limited to reading or reviewing clinical polysomnograms (CPSGs) and then writing reports based on them, reimbursement for which is on a fee-for-service basis. The fee may vary from 10% to 25% of the charge for the CPSG, and may be billed and collected separately or may be included as part of the overall charge for the CPSG by the hospital, which then pays the somnologist. Alternatively, the somnologist-medical director may have an office in the sleep center where patients are seen in a usual fee-for-service consultation practice with charges guided by complexity of the case, the length of contact, local custom, and agreements with managed care plans. A limited number of somnologists have established freestanding sleep centers, modeled after freestanding radiology offices, EEG laboratories, and dialysis centers. In these centers, all of the expenses are borne by the physician, who then bills for a total service. Customary fees in somnology reflect a level of remuneration commensurate with that of other psychiatric subspecialties. Psychiatrist-somnologists can devote a major portion of their time to sleep disorders to provide the core of their income or invest more limited time to the practice to provide supplemental income.

Legal Considerations

There are opportunities for somnologists to be involved with the legal system, as illustrated in the following two case examples:

> Mr. C, a 63-year-old man, was accused by his son's former wife of having molested his 14-year-old granddaughter. The accusation included a charge of penile penetration. Mr. C was sent to a sleep disorders center by his attorney. He claimed he was impotent and incapable of penetration. A sleep laboratory evaluation for nocturnal penile tumescence showed no evidence of tumescence on three nights of monitoring—a finding that supported Mr. C's claim of impotence.

> A young man, Mr. D, was reported in the newspapers to have awakened in the middle of night, driven across town, and physically assaulted and killed his mother-in-law. He was acquitted based largely on the testimony of several somnologists that he was in a somnambulistic state during the tragic episode and therefore was not responsible for his actions.

The practice of sleep disorders medicine opens practitioners to new potentials for extended medical liability. A patient with obstructive sleep apnea who develops irreversible cardiovascular changes because of inadequate treatment could initiate a malpractice suit. A sleepy patient who has an automobile accident that results in damage to person and property may well raise questions about the adequacy of diagnosis and treatment.

Concerns about legal liability are no greater in somnology than in the rest of medicine. Documentation of prudent evaluation and treatment of an informed patient with whom the physician remains in contact provides the best shield for physicians against charges of inadequate or inappropriate medical care. Certainly, psychiatrist-somnologists should ensure that their professional liability insurance covers this aspect of their practice.

Conclusion

The field of somnology is an open one; opportunities abound. Modern psychiatrists with a balanced background in the emotional and biological basis for illness are well prepared for training in sleep disorders medicine. Young or old, male or female, native or foreign born, all qualified psychiatric practitioners have an equal role in serving the patient with disorders of sleep.

References

American Sleep Disorders Association: The International Classification of Sleep Disorders: Diagnostic and Coding Manual. Lawrence, KS, Allen Press, 1990

Arkin AM, Antrobus JS, Ellman SJ (eds): The Mind in Sleep: Psychology and Psychophysiology. Hillsdale, NJ, Lawrence Erlbaum, 1978

Brunner J: The Acts of Meaning. Cambridge, MA, Harvard University Press, 1990

Aserinsky E, Kleitman N: Regularly occurring periods of eye motility and concomitant phenomena during sleep. Science 118:273–274, 1953

Cartwright R: A network of dreams, in Sleep and Cognition. Edited by Bootzin PR, Kihlstrom JF, Schacter DL. Washington, DC, American Psychological Association, 1990, pp 179–189

Chase MH, Lydic R, O'Connor C (eds): Sleep Research, Vols 1–23. Los Angeles, CA, UCLA Brain Information Service/Brain Research Institute, 1972–1990

Delaney G: Living Your Dreams. San Francisco, CA, Harper & Row, 1979

Dement WC, Kleitman N: Cyclic variations in EEG during sleep and their relation to eye movements, body motility, and dreaming. Electroencephalogr Clin Neurophysiol 9:673–690, 1957

Foulkes D: Dreaming: A Cognitive-Psychological Analysis. Hillsdale, NJ, Lawrence Erlbaum, 1985

Gastaut H, Tassinari CA, Duron B: Polygraphic study of the episodic diurnal and nocturnal manifestations of the Pickwick syndrome. Brain Res 2:167–186, 1966

Hathaway SR, McKinley JC: Minnesota Multiphasic Personality Inventory, Revised. Minneapolis, MN, University of Minnesota, 1970

Jung C: Approaching the unconscious, in Man and His Symbols. New York, Doubleday, 1964, pp 18–103

Kleitman N: Sleep and Wakefulness, 2nd Edition. Chicago, IL, University of Chicago Press, 1963

Kramer M: Obstructive sleep apnea—one night is not enough! Journal of Psychiatry and Related Sciences 17:205, 1988

Kramer M: The prediction of obstructive sleep apnea, in Sleep 88: Proceedings of the Ninth European Congress on Sleep Research, Jerusalem (Israel), September 4–9, 1988. Edited by Horne J. New York, Gustav Fischer Verlag, 1989, pp 256–259

Kramer M: Nightmares (dream disturbances) in post traumatic stress disorder: implications for a theory of dreaming, in Sleep and Cognition. Edited by Bootzin PR, Kihlstrom JF, Schacter DL. Washington, DC, American Psychological Association, 1990, pp 190–202

Kramer M: The selective mood regulatory function of dreaming: an update and revision, in The Functions of Dreaming. Edited by Moffitt AR, Kramer M, Hoffman RF. Albany, NY, State University of New York Press, 1993, pp 139–195

Kramer M, McGinnis W: Cataplexy—muscle weakness—McArdle's syndrome: a case report. Sleep Research 15:193, 1986

Kramer M, Roth T: Dream translation. Israel Annals of Psychiatry and Related Disciplines 15:336–351, 1977

Kryger MH, Roth T, Dement WC (eds): Principles and Practice of Sleep Medicine. Philadelphia, PA, WB Saunders, 1989

LaBerge S: Lucid Dreaming. Los Angeles, CA, Jeremy P. Tarcher, 1985

Mellinger GD, Balter MB, Uhlenhuth EH: Insomnia and its treatment: prevalence and correlates. Arch Gen Psychiatry 42:225–232, 1985

Moffitt AR, Kramer M, Hoffman RF (eds): The Functions of Dreaming. Albany, NY, State University of New York Press, 1993

Rechtschaffen A, Kales A (eds): A Manual of Standardized Terminology, Techniques and Scoring System for Sleep Stages of Human Subjects. Los Angeles, CA, UCLA Brain Information Service/Brain Research Institute, 1963

Reite ML, Nagel KE, Ruddy JR: Concise Guide to Evaluation and Management of Sleep Disorders. Washington, DC, American Psychiatric Press, 1990

States BO: Dreams and Story Telling. Ithaca, NY, Cornell University Press, 1993

Ullman M, Zimmerman N: Working With Dreams. Los Angeles, CA, Jeremy P. Tarcher, 1979

Section II:
Setting-Related Careers

Hospital-Based Practice

CHAPTER FIVE

Inpatient Psychiatry

Margaret J. Dorfman, M.D.
John J. Haggerty, Jr., M.D.

All psychiatrists, having completed psychiatric residency training, are more familiar with practice in inpatient settings than with any other practice site. At present, inpatient psychiatry is practiced in various settings, including general hospital psychiatric units (which may be affiliated with community mental health centers or residency training programs), state hospitals (on short-term or long-term units), and private hospitals. In this chapter, we discuss the history of inpatient mental hospitals, the advantages and disadvantages of hospital-based practice for psychiatrists, and the specific characteristics of each of these settings. We then look at the knowledge base needed for hospital-based practice, and at special considerations about hospital psychiatric practice for women, minorities, and international medical graduates. Finally, we offer predictions about the future of this specialty.

History of Inpatient Mental Hospitals

Inpatient psychiatry has had a long and checkered history that continues to influence contemporary practice. Those contemplating a career in this specialty will benefit from understanding its background.

In the United States, prior to the establishment of hospitals, mentally ill individuals at best were housed in jails, almshouses, and workhouses and at worst were allowed to drift from village to village or were auctioned off as laborers (Hall et al. 1944). Thus, the development of hospitals was seen as a charitable endeavor as well as a benefit to the community (Bell 1980).

In the first hospitals in Europe and the United States, the "insane" were kept chained in unheated and dirty cells (Bell 1980). Hospital conditions began to be improved with the "moral treatment" started by Philippe Pinel in France and William Tuke in England (Freedman et al. 1978), a movement that swept through Europe and reached this country when Benjamin Rush protested the conditions at the Pennsylvania Hospital (Hall et al. 1944).

By 1843, there were 24 public and private institutions for the mentally ill in the United States (Hall et al. 1944). In the years that followed, many more were built and the quality of care upgraded, largely through the crusading efforts of Dorothea Lynde Dix. By the 1800s, the tractable mentally ill were generally treated kindly, although agitated or violent patients were still restrained into immobility for long periods, threatened with physical punishment, and "treated" with techniques like dousing in cold water (Bell 1980). Advocacy by local reformers led to the development of laws for inspecting and regulating the institutions and stricter commitment laws (Bell 1980).

By the early 1900s, renewed emphasis was placed on active treatment, including the use of analytic therapy for psychotic patients (Bell 1980). Later, more effective biological treatments were developed, beginning with the shock therapies (insulin, pentylenetetrazol [Metrazol], and electroconvulsive treatment), which were curative for some patients but vastly overused and harmful to others. In 1952, chlorpromazine was introduced, followed by additional antipsychotic, antidepressant, and antimanic medications. Although not without significant side effects, these allowed many previously incurable patients to be treated and discharged.

At the same time that pharmacotherapy was transforming hospital psychiatry, the community psychiatry movement was having at least as great an impact. Community psychiatry advocates saw hospitalization in a state institution as inherently negative, causing inertia and dependency in patients, stigmatizing them, and isolating them from their family and community (Bell 1980).

In 1961, the federal Joint Commission on Mental Illness and Mental Health published "Action for Mental Health," a report advocating community-based care with inpatient services in psychiatric units of general hospitals. In 1963, President John F. Kennedy signed the Community Mental Health Act, which began the push for deinstitutionalization. Between 1955 and 1970, there was an average reduction of 33% in the number of patients housed in institutions (Bell 1980).

Problems soon became apparent. The community system, lacking complete services like housing and vocational rehabilitation, could not meet the needs of discharged patients; in addition, ostracism and fear of mentally ill individuals were still commonplace (Bell 1980). More recently, concern about mentally ill homeless individuals and "revolving door" patients has become widespread. As a result, long-term hospitalization has again become recognized as a necessary treatment modality for some patients, yet funding for this option continues to decrease in many states (Bell 1980).

At the same time that state hospitals were shrinking or closing, general hospital psychiatric units were multiplying. In addition, private psychiatric hospitals, many owned by proprietary chains, became widespread as a result of improved insurance coverage of treatment of mental illness. More recently, psychiatric units have been shrinking or closing as rates, admissions, and lengths of stay have been more and more closely monitored by third-party payers under managed care.

Advantages and Disadvantages of Hospital-Based Psychiatry

Although no two careers in inpatient psychiatry are alike, the sources of satisfaction and dissatisfaction are similar across the spectrum.

Advantages

Inpatient work provides rich clinical experience. A greater range of clinical cases are encountered on inpatient units than elsewhere, including rare and complicated disorders that provide invigorating intellectual challenges. Although patients' lengths of stay have certainly shortened significantly, there are still opportunities to treat patients more intensively, combining somatic, dynamic, group, and family treatment in a synergistic effort often not feasible for non-hospitalized patients. Some particularly powerful and gratifying forms of treatment, such as electroconvulsive therapy (ECT) or aggressive pharmacotherapy, can often be provided safely only in hospital settings. Inpatient psychiatrists also have the satisfaction of helping large numbers of patients and of seeing clear-cut improvement in many patients in a relatively brief time.

Inpatient work also offers the opportunity to work as part of a team rather than in isolation. One has daily interaction with psychiatric and nonpsychiatric medical colleagues. Difficult decisions can be shared and discussed with clinical team members. Most hospitals also offer opportunities for continuing education. By being part of an administrative team, a psychiatrist can have the exciting experience of shaping treatment programs and facility design.

The most frequently mentioned advantage of inpatient work is a practical one: the potential for generating stable income. Whereas it may take years for independent outpatient-based psychiatrists to develop a viable referral network, hospital-based psychiatrists can more readily fill their practice by virtue of access to patients needing immediate and intensive treatment. Third-party reimbursement is also more certain for brief inpatient treatment than for outpatient treatment.

Disadvantages

Inpatient psychiatry clearly has a high "burnout" rate, with many psychiatrists, once established, electing not to continue this type of work.

Although managed care has left no area of clinical practice untouched, it probably impacts the life of the inpatient psychiatrist to a greater extent than others; limiting hospital utilization is priority number one of all managed care contractors. The administrative time drain on inpatient practitioners can be considerable. Inpatient psychiatrists can expect to spend a minimum of 15–30 minutes of unbillable time per patient per week talking with reviewers. More importantly, the ability to engage in meaningful treatment planning has been significantly disrupted by arbitrary black box decisions that make lengths of stay highly unpredictable (Schreter 1993). Some hospital settings have been able to offset this arbitrariness by constructing stable and consistent partnerships with a single managed care contractor. Yet, even in these hospitals, inpatient psychiatrists must tolerate constant intrusions on their clinical work and questioning of their judgment.

In addition to time demands involved in responding to outside reviewers, inpatient psychiatrists must also be involved in hospital utilization and quality assurance processes. All of this means that psychiatrists in inpatient settings must struggle with administrative time taken away from patient care, intrusiveness into patient confidentiality and physician judgment, and ethical conflicts generated by having to cut costs while trying to furnish needed treatment. Clearly, this is a major source of stress.

Other intrinsic factors also impact the quality of life for inpatient psychiatrists. Intense exposure to very sick patients, including those requiring involuntary treatment, can erode a caregiver's sense of well-being and confidence. Rapid patient turnover rates engender feelings of discontinuity and disorganization. A hospital-based clinician has to manage not only patients' treatment but the feelings of other hospital staff members. It can be difficult to plan schedules because of the unpredictability of admissions and ward crises. Because there are likely to be on-call responsibilities, planning of day-to-day work as well as coverage while away can be problematic.

It is fortunate for patients that many inpatient psychiatrists find that the satisfactions of this kind of work outweigh the disadvantages. Because the satisfactions and disadvantages vary by type of practice, we now look at some of these settings in greater depth.

Different Settings for Hospital-Based Psychiatry

General Hospital Psychiatry

Whereas many psychiatrists include treatment of inpatients in one or more general hospitals as part of their work, some choose to do this exclusively. At present, a general hospital psychiatrist can usually earn a good living with this kind of practice. It is rare for there to be a prolonged "drought" period in patient hospitalizations and consultations. If the physician is careful to treat only those with third-party coverage and to follow insurers' guidelines regarding precertification and length-of-stay approval, payment is regularly forthcoming. Generally, physicians can choose to accept emergency admissions or not, except perhaps when on call for their group or unit, and they can find other attendings who are willing to cover their patients to allow for vacation. This time off, however, is unpaid, so physicians must balance financial needs against needs for education, recreation, and relaxation. In addition, general hospital psychiatrists must generally provide for their own benefits, including health and malpractice insurance.

Psychiatrists' duties are those that are familiar to any resident. Newly admitted patients must have psychiatric and physical evaluations and orders must be written. Psychiatrists need to attend treatment team meetings, which are usually brief and timed to be fairly convenient. Daily interviews with patients after admission are generally mandated, as are daily and weekend notes for Medicaid and Medicare patients and increasingly so for others as well, depending on hospital bylaws and insurance requirements. Follow-up care must be arranged and discharge summaries dictated.

Night and weekend on-call responsibilities vary considerably, depending on the hospital. In some cases, all attendings on staff rotate call; in others, attendings establish groups and arrange to cross-cover each other. Nighttime admission of medically or psychiatrically unstable patients requires expeditious evaluation, but hospital bylaws often allow for evaluation of more stable patients the following day.

State Hospital Psychiatry

The duties of a state hospital psychiatrist will depend both on the quality of the hospital and on the type of ward assignment. The number of patients a psychiatrist is responsible for is generally proportional to the chronicity of their illness. On an acute ward, a physician may have as few as 12 patients or as many as 30. With treatment-resistant chronic patients, the caseload would usually be at least 50 patients and often more.

Work on a state hospital acute ward is similar to that on a general hospital psychiatric unit, though the patient population differs. Adult patients in a general hospital unit have most often been admitted for mood disorders, often complicated by dementia, character pathology, or substance abuse. Adult patients in state hospitals have most often been admitted for exacerbations of schizophrenia or mania, though severely depressed patients are not uncommon. State hospital patients are more likely to be severely ill and may require intrusive measures, such as seclusion, restraint, or forced medication. Despite the severity of their illness, however, many respond well to treatment and can be discharged fairly rapidly. Psychiatrists treating such patients must be expert in the use of psychotropic medications. They may also provide individual therapy; because of time pressures, sessions are less frequent and shorter than on a general hospital unit.

Work on a state hospital chronic unit is quite different from that on an acute unit. In a chronic unit, each patient's progress will be slower and the goals more modest. Psychiatrists have few admissions and, over time, get to know their patients well. The primary interventions for these patients often become nonmedical and may be the responsibility of health care providers other than psychiatrists. Psychiatrists primarily monitor symptoms and provide pharmacotherapy, and may also be responsible for supervising the other providers. Chronic patients are seen less often than are acutely ill ones, with significantly fewer note-writing requirements; life for both psychiatrists and patients is slower paced.

State hospital positions are salaried, with paid vacations and sick leave, and generally have personal and professional insurance provided. Extra pay may also be provided for on-call time. Because of the need to fill physician vacancies in state hospitals, salaries have become more competitive in recent years. In addition, many states provide continuing medical education directly or allow physician leave time to obtain it.

Night and weekend on-call duty may be rotated among the staff, contracted out, or provided through some combination of these. If on-call responsibility is not contracted out, there is typically some type of compensation given for this service, either in time or money. On-call times are likely to be busy, because new admissions will generally need to be evaluated and treated rapidly because of the severity of their condition.

Mental Health Center Inpatient Psychiatry

In most cases, mental health center psychiatrists combine inpatient and outpatient responsibilities, but some care only for hospitalized patients. Their work has much in common with both state and general hospital psychiatry.

Typically, a mental health center inpatient unit is located in a general hospital and arranges with a state hospital for the transfer of patients who are extremely or persistently violent. The unit is a locked ward allowing for the care of moderately violent patients as well as other less agitated schizophrenic, manic, and depressed patients. Patients who abuse substances are also admitted there for detoxification.

Mental health center inpatient psychiatrists can expect many admissions and readmissions of severely ill patients for short stays. Psychotropic medication management is essential, but, for some patients, psychotherapy is equally important. Requirements for frequency of interviews and notes are the same as those of a general hospital and, therefore, likely to be stringent.

Because there are usually just one or two psychiatrists responsible for the unit, arrangements are often made to ease the burdens of night and weekend call by using emergency room physicians for initial evaluations and physical examinations, with a psychiatrist available by telephone, or by hiring "moonlighting" psychiatrists to provide weekend care.

Because of recruitment problems, salaries for mental health center inpatient psychiatrists may be competitive or even generous, depending on funding sources. Additional compensation for on-call time is often included. Vacation and sick leave are provided, as are medical insurance and other benefits.

Private Hospital Psychiatry

Despite changes attributable to the managed care system, private hospital psychiatry still tends to be more lucrative and in some ways more relaxed than inpatient psychiatry elsewhere. Many proprietary chains hire physicians and pay them very generous salaries for at least a year or two until they become established. Other perks tend to be included, such as rent-free offices and time off to see outpatients. There are generous benefit packages, including, of course, vacation and sick leave.

Depending on the hospital's financial status, staffing may be generous or lean. Owners, administrators, and policies can change rapidly, especially if the hospital is having financial difficulties; these can lead to shifts in physicians' job conditions and satisfaction. This is true for other staff members as well, and there can be rapid turnover of staff. Of additional concern is the potential for ethical pitfalls and conflicts of interest, which can arise from the expectation that patients will be hospitalized at the one hospital providing salary and perks.

As is true for general hospital psychiatrists, private hospital psychiatrists are responsible for meeting third-party payer requirements for precertification and justification of length of stay. They must also adhere to hospital policies, which may include required psychological or complex diagnostic procedures on all newly admitted patients, and answer to hospital administrators, whose first concern is often cost and income.

Patients admitted to private hospitals have diagnoses similar to those admitted to general hospital units. The psychiatrist is responsible for individual therapy and pharmacotherapy, and must interview patients daily, with a daily (including weekend) note required for most.

On-call responsibilities are usually rotated between staff members, though at times other physicians may be paid to help cover nights and weekends. Hospital policies often allow evaluations to take place the morning following a nighttime admission unless a patient's condition dictates otherwise.

Academic Inpatient Psychiatry

Inpatient unit positions are frequently assigned as an entry-level task for junior faculty. The academician–inpatient psychiatrist assumes overall responsibility for a number of patients, but because of the presence of residents, is a step removed from direct therapeutic involvement. Work hours are reasonable, but the draining and unpredictable nature of service commitments may interfere with concurrent teaching and, particularly, research activity, which may then impede professional advancement. Allowance for adequate "off service" time is highly desirable.

Salaries vary considerably, from low to generous. Personal and professional insurance are provided, as are vacation, sick leave, and continuing educational opportunities. The attending is often required to share in supervision of residents who cover nights and weekends.

Prerequisites for Inpatient Psychiatry

Currently there are no special certification requirements for practicing inpatient psychiatry, although there is some movement toward setting up minimum competency requirements for certain components, such as ECT.

Expert diagnostic skills. Inpatient psychiatrists must be expert diagnosticians. They must maintain the ability to assess and treat both physical and psychiatric disorders, including those physical disorders that manifest with psychiatric symptoms, given that the decision to admit a patient is often influenced by the coexistence of physical illnesses and psychiatric disorders. In addition to their expertise with both acute and chronic psychiatric disorders, inpatient psychiatrists must also have some expertise in the diagnosis and treatment of substance abuse and geriatric disorders, because patients with a dual diagnosis and elderly patients are common in hospitals.

Familiarity with various treatment modalities. Inpatient psychiatrists must be comfortable with the use of all somatic psychiatric treatments, including all available psychopharmacological agents and ECT.

Knowledge of applicable legal considerations. Inpatient psychiatrists must know the commitment laws and laws and regulations concerning involuntary treatment applicable in their jurisdiction.

Ability to work as team member. An inpatient psychiatrist must be able to effectively interact with and lead a multidisciplinary team. Even the most gifted physicians will be able to ensure good treatment only if they are able to convey treatment principles to staff and organize, support, and focus the efforts of those who will be working with patients the other 23 hours of the day. Comfort with delegating responsibilities is essential, as is the ability to perceive and influence group process and countertransference.

Special Considerations

Hospital psychiatry has some particularly relevant advantages for women, minorities, and international medical graduates.

Inpatient practice provides early income and acquaintance with a number of patients, physicians, and staff members. The quality of a psychiatrist's work is visible to others, and thus the physician can establish a reputation for professional competence. If the psychiatrist's goal is to develop a mixed practice of inpatients and outpatients, following discharged patients will help build the outpatient component of his or her practice. Advancement to unit leadership can be a first step into administrative psychiatry.

Many positions are salaried for a fixed number of hours per week, including part-time work. Fee-for-service work can be limited, with a small patient load and no emergency admissions. On-call responsibilities are known in advance and generally limited.

Future Developments

The last half-century has seen unprecedented changes in the nature of psychiatric hospitals, and the pace of change continues to be rapid. Several developments are particularly likely to affect the future development of inpatient psychiatry.

First, market competition and emphasis on cost-of-service delivery are pushing psychiatric inpatient units into developing special niches in which they can operate most efficiently. Thus, psychiatrists may less often work in general units and more often focus on a specific subset of the psychiatric population (e.g., geriatric patients, chemical dependency patients, depressed patients). Inpatient psychiatric stays are likely to continue to shorten, with growing reliance on alternatives to hospitalization, such as day treatment, nonhospital residential centers, and respite homes that allow lower staffing levels and fewer certification requirements. At the same time, there is growing recognition of the need for extended institutionalization for a small number of chronically ill patients. Continuing changes in health care financing, including changes in the ways physicians' services are compensated, are sure to have an—as yet unpredictable—impact on inpatient care.

Further, psychiatrists can also anticipate that there will be significant changes in the nature of psychiatric inpatient populations in the near future. Two developments are particularly noteworthy. The first is the current epidemic of acquired immunodeficiency syndrome (AIDS); because of the prevalence of dementia associated with this syndrome, the burden of caring for patients with AIDS may fall increasingly on the shoulders of inpatient psychiatrists. This may call for existing and future units to develop new capabilities to handle combined neuropsychiatric and medical illnesses. Second, the shifting age distribution of the United States population toward an increasingly elderly population will require the development of improved geriatric psychiatry services over the next half-century.

Finally, it is likely that, with continued technological development, inpatient psychiatrists will have to handle new and more complex diagnostic and treatment tools requiring relatively higher degrees of technological sophistication.

Some of the specifics of services provided by inpatient psychiatrists will undoubtedly be altered. Many would hope that current review and payment procedures will change. What will not change in the foreseeable future is the need for psychiatrists to treat the desperately ill population seen in hospital-based settings.

References

Bell LV: Treating the Mentally Ill. New York, Praeger, 1980
Community Mental Health Act of 1963, Public Law 88-164
Freedman AM, Kaplan HI, Sadock BJ (eds): Comprehensive Textbook of Psychiatry/II. Baltimore, MD, Williams & Wilkins, 1978

Hall JU, Zilhouse G, Bunker HA (eds): One Hundred Years of American Psychiatry. New York, Columbia University Press, 1944

Joint Commission on Mental Illness and Mental Health: Report to Congress: Action for Mental Health. New York, Basic Books, 1961

Schreter RK: Ten trends in managed care and their impact on the biopsychosocial model. Hosp Community Psychiatry 44:325–327, 1993

For Further Reading

Olelen KW, Johnson MP: A "facilitated" model of inpatient psychiatric care. Hosp Community Psychiatry 44:879–882, 1993

CHAPTER SIX

Emergency Psychiatry

Gail M. Barton, M.D., M.P.H.

A career in emergency psychiatry is for those who enjoy surprises, excitement, diagnostic challenges, and decisions in a pressure-cooker environment.

Historical Considerations

Emergency psychiatry is a relatively young field. As yet, it is not a subspecialty with board examinations, but there currently is interest in seeking subspecialty status for it. Forty years ago, emergency psychiatry was not a separate endeavor from general psychiatry. State mental hospitals provided long-term care for the majority of patients, and those who were considered to need care were simply brought to their admitting units. By the 1950s, with the more open-door policies of state hospitals and the introduction of psychotropic medications, lengths of stay for patients had decreased and repeated admissions had become more commonplace.

The community mental health center (CMHC) movement of the 1960s created facilities to serve the mentally ill in the community; an adjunct development was the establishment of psychiatric emergency components such as 24-hour telephone answering services, crisis walk-in services, and aftercare capability. Care for psychiatric emergencies became more focused around community resources and less around state mental hospital facilities. This led to more patients presenting to community hospital emergency rooms and on the doorsteps of the community mental health centers. At first the hospitals and the CMHCs operated in isolation from one another. Increasingly, however, they came to appreciate the fact that by joining forces they could provide more adequate medical screening to the CMHC clientele and outreach capability to general hospital emergency departments (Zealberg et al. 1993).

General Description of the Work and the Setting

The Nature of Emergency Psychiatry

In the past, only one question had to be answered in connection with emergency psychiatry practice: Is it safe to let the patient go or does the patient need to be admitted? Now emergency psychiatrists must deal with more complex issues than simply the commitment issue, which in and of itself has become more complicated. The answers to the following four questions give an indication of what emergency psychiatry currently entails:

1. What situations are considered psychiatric emergencies?
2. Where are psychiatric emergencies handled?
3. When do psychiatric emergencies occur?
4. Who handles psychiatric emergencies?

What situations are considered psychiatric emergencies? Who decides if there is a psychiatric emergency, and what defines such an emergency? The American Psychiatric Association (APA) Task Force on Psychiatric Emergency Care Issues studied this issue from 1978 to 1983 and evolved the following definition of a *psychiatric emergency:*

> An acute disturbance of thought, mood, behavior or social relationship that requires an immediate intervention as defined by the patient, the family or the community. (Barton et al. 1983, p. 25)

Where are psychiatric emergencies handled? The answer is in the "field" or community by the police, citizens, or paramedics or emergency medical technicians, or in the community health centers, general hospitals, or, less often, state hospital facilities (Zealberg et al. 1992).

When do psychiatric emergencies occur? The "when" of psychiatric emergencies is anytime, day or night.

Who handles psychiatric emergencies? Any mental health professional may deal with psychiatric emergencies, including a psychiatrist or a psychiatric resident. Most psychiatrists are introduced to emergency psychiatry in a very unpalatable manner: by being assigned to cover emergency psychiatry call nights and weekends as soon as they start their residency. Who better to do the job? Almost anyone with more experience!

Description of Emergency Psychiatry

The important tasks in emergency psychiatry practice are to find out what the patient is complaining of, what the patient needs, and what resources are available. Residents soon learn that on nights and weekends, admitting a patient may be all that is possible because other resources may be closed after 5:00 P.M. and on weekends. The more comprehensive psychiatric emergency services have holding beds so that individuals can be monitored for up to 72 hours in the service (Forster 1993; Sherman 1993). In these cases, the role of the emergency psychiatrist is expanded to more of a treatment and management orientation rather than an evaluation and diagnostic one.

Work Conditions

Even though emergency care is a 24-hour service, many sites still do not have full-time positions available for emergency psychiatrists and merely add night and weekend call duties to the regular work weeks of their existing staff psychiatrists. Some emergency service psychiatrists may even take calls from home, whereas others stay on site for their shifts.

State, public, and private hospitals, as well as academic institutions, may hire psychiatrists or moonlighting psychiatrists-in-training to run their emergency psychiatry departments during off hours (Strout 1991). Others may have sufficient business to hire psychiatrists for regular weekday hours. If the latter situation exists, the nighttime and weekend schedules are usually filled through rotation of duties between daytime psychiatrists or through affiliation with a group who takes calls.

The salary for an emergency psychiatrist depends on the practice setting. Academia generally pays less well than private hospitals. A part-time, add-on, salaried emergency psychiatrist earns well, but usually not enough to support a family. Big cities can offer high-paying jobs, but the high caseload can also cause burnout in a matter of months. The prospect of hundreds of patients to be screened in a big general hospital emergency department on each shift with few possible dispositions other than medicating and holding patients for a few days may not be appealing.

On the other hand, others may not wish to practice emergency psychiatry in a rural setting, where one often has to rely on the telephone and on patching resources together because distance and weather may prevent patients from reaching emergency rooms or resources may be nonexistent (Barton 1992). Patching a disposition together by using police, relatives, and local general practitioners may be all one can do until transportation to a definitive facility is feasible. In rural areas, it may take as long as several hours for screeners from local mental health centers to come to the assistance of a psychiatrist with a patient needing commitment because of the distance, other professional demands on their time, or different after-hours priorities.

Challenges Facing Emergency Psychiatrists

Frustrations and Disadvantages

Nature of patient population. Emergency psychiatry would be a pleasant and rewarding job if patients in emergency rooms were appreciative of psychiatrists' efforts, but much of the time they are not. Patients may ignore or deny their symptoms and leave the covering psychiatrist to use the powers of threatened commitment, medications, or restraints to keep them long enough to figure out if it would be safer to have them stay or go. Of course there are times when the emergency psychiatrist-in-training is able to lessen the distress of patients and families who present in emergency services or to find dispositions that fit their needs well.

Lack of patient follow-up. Another frustration for the emergency psychiatrist is not knowing what becomes of patients he or she has evaluated in the emergency department. Was the diagnosis the best and most accurate for that patient? Was the decision correct to send a patient home? Did the family really go into treatment? Did the neuroleptic given cause dystonia? Did the judge concur with the request for commitment? Did the receiving hospital keep the patient? Did the patient show up the next day for evaluation?

Attitudes of other emergency caregivers. Psychiatrists in an emergency service are confronted with the frequently disdainful attitude of other emergency team members toward patients, as if they believe that "if patients aren't bleeding, they are taking up valuable emergency room space"; if a psychiatrist needs to spend 2 hours talking to patients and their families, the patients are "wasting valuable time"; if they say angry or unintelligible things, "they are disturbing the emergency room team and the 'real' patients." Emergency psychiatrists end up fighting the stigma of mental illness, acting as advocates for patients' welfare, and wondering why the system of mental health care is so disconnected and often hostile. Because emergency care is the interface between the community and helping agencies, emergency psychiatrists see the warts of the system and of the people tending it.

One helpful way of managing the more negative staff attitudes is to hold case conferences about the problematic cases so that transferential attitudes can be addressed and modified over the long run. The roles of systems changer and patient evaluator are similar to those required by a typical consultation-liaison service.

Strenuous work conditions. Then there are the long hours, intensity of patient illnesses, overwhelming presentations, and frustrating lack of resources, all of which make burnout in psychiatric emergency service staff not uncommon. Many say that emergency psychiatry is a specialty for the young because the pace is so intense. On the other hand, experience is very helpful in dealing with a complex case or situation. Others will say a reason to go into emergency psychiatry is to organize a poorly run field.

Advantages

Exciting and gratifying work. As emergency psychiatry has become more legitimized and better organized, practitioners have increasingly come to view it as an interesting and attractive subspecialty. Many who practice emergency psychiatry are drawn by its challenges and excitement, an enthusiasm shared with others on the emergency team ("A Highly Visible Crisis Intervention Team," 1985). Who would want to miss the excitement and challenge of seeing if one can make the system work so that the alcoholic patient is accepted into a detoxification program, the mentally retarded patient with a broken leg receives orthopedic attention, the elderly woman who can no longer care for herself is accepted into a nursing home, the police allow the patient to surrender peacefully rather than to shoot the responding emergency psychiatrist or himself, the deeply depressed individual is convinced of the importance of hospital admission, or the schizophrenic patient receives psychotropic medication to dampen the threatening voices? One is met with a large variety of challenges regarding behavioral presentations of the patients, difficult differential diagnoses, challenging and complex disposition plan needs, and working as a member of a team in a pressure-cooker environment.

Diagnostic challenges. One of the major challenges of emergency psychiatry is figuring out what is really wrong with the patient. Does the patient have a medical problem that has been missed, like pneumonia rather than depression? Severe anemia rather than cantankerousness? A broken leg rather than hysteria? Family crises offer different challenges: the adolescent may have overdosed to signal that help is needed for the dysfunctional family; a rape victim may be blamed by the family for somehow inviting the attack, so that all family members need attention, care, and education; a schizophrenic mother who sees her children as instruments of the devil must be treated and her children protected.

Making the system work. A particular challenge for emergency psychiatrists is to get different health and mental health agencies to work together to assist in necessary dispositions for patients. For example, once the psychiatrist diagnoses a patient, social services may be willing to give emergency monetary aid if a temporary shelter is willing to take the patient in.

Schedule flexibility. Emergency psychiatry can now be practiced full-time in some settings and can be scheduled so as not to interfere with family, leisure, and recreation time as much as in some other sub-specialties of psychiatry.

Abundance of opportunities. The field of emergency psychiatry is still young; this provides the advantage of having the opportunity to develop standards, influence policy, teach good care, and initiate careful research by being involved at this pivotal time. It is also a field in which limitations because of race, sex, or ethnic origin are minimal because of the need for people to fill positions and the variety of settings in which positions are available (e.g., inner-city environments, Native American reservations, suburban settings); people in crisis want help. What counts the most is that an emergency psychiatrist be a caring and skilled professional.

Training

The ability to make the quick and complex decisions that are part of emergency psychiatry comes with training and experience. Formal training starts as a resident. Early on, one learns how scared and vulnerable one can feel with little training or authority but with great responsibility. Training should include instruction in a biopsychosocial philosophical framework, assessment and history taking, differential diagnosis, crisis intervention, short-term treatment, pharmacotherapy, disposition planning, case management, team work, handling of violence, managing a case in the community, record keeping, follow-up, continuity of care, legal and ethical considerations, consultation and liaison with other specialties and agencies, and understanding of managed care.

Many residents are forced to learn on the job, preferably with supervision by more senior residents or staff. Other training besides supervision on the job includes reviewing the literature related to emergency psychiatry; attending grand rounds; attending journal clubs that have emergency psychiatry as their focus; taking a shift with the police, emergency medical technicians, or a CMHC emergency crisis outreach worker; and attending special lectures on the handling of violence and on ethical and legal issues (Zealberg et al. 1990).

On-site supervision on a case-by-case basis in the early phases of training is preferable to supervision that is obtained the next morning after a hectic night of assessing patients and deciding what to do. It is unfortunate that staffing in most training sites is insufficient for night shifts but not for day shifts. In many residencies, first- and second-year residents take emergency calls; at some sites, more senior residents also take calls. It is preferable that more senior residents fulfill this responsibility. At that stage in training, the job seems less onerous because dispositions are better understood, connections with other care providers and agencies are better accomplished, and differential diagnoses are more in hand. The senior resident can also incorporate much-enjoyed supervision of the more junior residents.

Consultation-liaison work further prepares one for the complex dilemmas that other specialties face, and for dealing with staff attitudes, misunderstandings, and the stigma expressed toward the mentally ill. Community mental health rotations prepare a psychiatrist for going on home visits to evaluate crisis situations, for evaluating seriously and dangerously mentally ill individuals, and for working as a team member among different agencies. Some residencies provide a practicum on staff safety and the handling of violent individuals rather than ignoring the fact that there is a need to worry about safety. Requirements for residency program accreditation include emergency psychiatry training.

Opportunities and Responsibilities

A new organization—the American Association of Emergency Psychiatrists—has been formed to provide networking, support, and consistency in the practice of emergency psychiatry. Prior to this, the APA appointed a Task Force on Emergency Psychiatric Issues, which spent a great deal of time documenting the state of the art and the problems, preparing a set of standards, and developing monographs (Barton and Friedman 1986; Bassuk et al. 1983; Comstock et al. 1984; Farley et al. 1979; Fauman and Fauman 1981; Gorton and Partridge 1982; Slaby et al. 1981; Soreff 1981), as well as organizing regional and national workshops to increase awareness and expertise in this area. Consequently, there is growing awareness of emergency psychiatry as an emerging subspecialty of psychiatry. The American Board of Psychiatry and Neurology now solicits examination questions on emergency psychiatry; the APA's Psychiatric Knowledge and Skills Assessment Program, PKSAP-VI, includes one whole section on emergency psychiatry; and the American College of Psychiatrists' Psychiatric Residents-in-Training Examination has questions relating to emergency psychiatry.

The Joint Commission on the Accreditation of Healthcare Organizations expects quality management audits of cases in the emergency department, including having residents' cases being audited by senior staff. Such legitimization and oversight of emergency psychiatry is gratifying. This field is increasingly becoming one with standards of care, rather than one where the level of care is determined simply by the skills of the provider (Sherman 1993). Psychiatrists now running psychiatric emergency services are more likely to have been trained in emergency psychiatry than to have just been assigned there without specific training. There is also an expanding body of literature and increased research efforts in emergency psychiatry (Hillard 1990; Mezzich and Zimmer 1991).

As emergency medicine has continued to become a formalized specialty over the past 30 years, emergency psychiatry also has expanded and matured to provide full-time opportunities. It is a far cry from the analyst's couch and as such appeals to those psychiatrists who wish to remain much closer to general medicine. Emergency psychiatry also has kinship to inpatient psychiatry because of the rapid turnaround time in evaluating patients, the crisis nature of treatment, and the procedures of selecting the best provisional disposition. Its similarity to consultation-liaison psychiatry is so close that often emergency psychiatrists find themselves fulfilling this role on nights and weekends at many sites as well.

Legal Considerations

A large number of legal issues challenge emergency psychiatrists, as the emergency room constitutes the boundary between society and the hospital, between being labeled healthy or sick, between being diagnosed competent or incompetent, between being in need of care or not. The emergency psychiatrist must decide the following issues, among others:

- Whether a patient should be hospitalized and, if so, voluntarily or with the involvement of the court
- Whether a patient has the right to treatment or the right to refuse treatment
- Whether society would be jeopardized by the release of a patient
- Whether a patient legitimately lost the prescribed medication or is trying to manipulate information for the sake of feeding an addiction
- Whether confidentiality should be breached because a patient is threatening to kill someone
- Whether a significant other should be called for information about an unconscious patient
- Whether an examining room door should be left open for the treating team's safety, even though that means threatening the patient's confidentiality
- Whether a patient should be restrained from leaving because a life-threatening illness may underlie the presenting agitation
- Which environment would be the least restrictive to the bizarrely acting patient, yet secure enough that the patient receives the needed treatment (e.g., a jail, state hospital, detoxification center, shelter)

References

A highly visible crisis intervention team: the Emergency Crisis Intervention Team, McLean County Center for Human Services, Bloomington, Illinois. Hosp Community Psychiatry 36:1213–1214, 1985

Barton GM: The practice of emergency psychiatry in rural areas. Hosp Community Psychiatry 43:965–967, 1992

Barton GM, Friedman RS (eds): Handbook of Emergency Psychiatry for Clinical Administrators. New York, Haworth Press, 1986

Barton GM, Slaby A, Fauman B, et al: Task Force Report (Draft) on Psychiatric Emergency Care Issues. Washington, DC, American Psychiatric Association, 1983

Bassuk EL, Fox S, Pendergast KJ: Behavioral Emergencies: A Field Guide for EMTs and Paramedics. Boston, MA, Little, Brown, 1983

Comstock B, Fann E, Pokornoy A, et al: The Phenomenology and Treatment of Psychiatric Emergencies. Jamaica, NY, Spectrum, 1984

Farley GK, Eckhardt LO, Hebert FB: Handbook of Child and Adolescent Psychiatric Emergencies. New York, Wiley, 1979

Fauman BJ, Fauman M: Emergency Psychiatry for the House Officer. Baltimore, MD, Williams & Wilkins, 1981

Forster P: Innovative programs in an urban psychiatric emergency service. Paper presented at the annual meeting of the American Association of General Hospital Psychiatrists, Boston, MA, June 19, 1993

Gorton JG, Partridge R (eds): Practice and Management of Psychiatric Emergency Care. St. Louis, MO, CV Mosby, 1982

Hillard JR (ed): Manual of Clinical Emergency Psychiatry. Washington, DC, American Psychiatric Press, 1990

Mezzich JE, Zimmer B (eds): Emergency Psychiatry. Madison, CT, International Universities Press, 1991

Sherman C: 72-hour ER stay helps predict violence. Clinical Psychiatry News 21:1, 12, June 1993

Slaby AE, Lieb J, Tancredi LR: A Handbook of Psychiatric Emergencies, 2nd Edition. Garden City, NY, Medical Examination Publishing, 1981

Soreff S: Management of the Psychiatric Emergency. New York, Wiley, 1981

Strout BA: Profiles of psychiatric crisis response systems, community support program. Rockville, MD, National Institute of Mental Health, 1991

Zealberg JJ, Santos AB, Hiers TB, et al: From the benches to the trenches: training residents to provide emergency outreach services—a public/academic project. Academic Psychiatry 14:211–217, 1990

Zealberg JJ, Christie SD, Puckett JA, et al: A mobile crisis program: collaboration between emergency psychiatric services and police. Hosp Community Psychiatry 43:612–615, 1992

Zealberg J, Santos AB, Fisher R: Benefits of mobile crisis programs. Hosp Community Psychiatry 44:16–17, 1993

CHAPTER SEVEN

Consultation-Liaison Psychiatry

Thomas N. Wise, M.D.
Miriam B. Rosenthal, M.D.

Introduction

Consultation-liaison psychiatry is the clinical derivative of psychosomatic medicine. It is the practice of psychiatry within a medical care system for both hospitalized and ambulatory patients. This psychiatric specialty is defined by its specific patient population—those who are or think they are medically ill—and thus includes a diverse range of patients in a variety of settings.

Psychosomatic is an inherently vague term; it connotes a linear causality that is philosophically untenable from a methodological point of view (McHugh and Slavney 1983). Although the term was first used by Heinroth in 1843, the interrelationship between mind and body has been an enduring concept since the birth of modern civilization. Galen, using Aristotle's concepts of causality in biological phenomena, emphasized a multifactorial approach in understanding illness (Siegel 1973). Famous physicians frequently cited the effects of emotions on bodily function. Francis Bacon urged investigation of physical illness from a perspective of interactionism with psychological phenomena, whereas William Harvey, the cardiovascular anatomist, wrote about the influence of emotional events on bodily functions (Hunter and Macalpine 1963). Although Cartesian dualism has been cited as a provocateur of splitting mind from body, Brown (1985) argued that Descartes' psychological approach allowed a different method of study rather than dualistic thinking. Serious students of psychosomatic medicine should review the works of Lipowski (1985) and Weiner (1977) for a history of this branch of medicine.

Thus, although psychiatrists have long been interested in theoretical approaches to physical illness, it was only when psychiatric physicians entered the general medical arena (i.e., hospitals) that consultation psychiatry was born. This branch of psychiatry involves direct clinical care, education of both psychiatric and nonpsychiatric physicians, and a variety of research endeavors, including studies of the psychological aspects of care and health service questions such as cost-effective management. Although it traditionally has been based in hospitals, with the evolution of family medicine, consultation psychiatry has moved to office settings. In liaison work, the psychiatrist is based and probably works mostly in a department other than psychiatry. The consultant-liaison psychiatrist often practices in other settings as well (e.g., general outpatient psychiatry).

Nature of the Practice

Consultation psychiatrists' main clinical duty is that denoted by the title of their subspecialty—seeing patients in consultation with other physicians. Consultation work in medical settings differs from consultation to social agencies in that consultant physicians remain part of a medical culture (Strain and Grossman 1974). There are a wide variety of clinical conditions for which consultations are requested.

Although various models have been proposed for the process of psychiatric consultation, the most useful approach is a patient-centered consultation where a diagnosis is made and treatment recommendations are communicated to the consultee, a process delineated by Meyer and Mendelson (1961). Specifically, the consultee-physician's uncertainty regarding a certain patient's condition generates a consultation request. The consulting psychiatrist then becomes the leader of a small group composed of patient, treating staff, physician, and other members of a patient's treatment team. Once this small group evolves and the psychiatrist conducts the formal interview and follow-up visits with the group, tensions within the group regarding the patient frequently diminish as the consultation clarifies the patient's difficulties. Thus, Meyer and Mendelson's approach is important because it provides an explanation both of the process of consultation work and of how consultation can be an exciting clinical experience. This intellectual understanding helps allay various aspects of burnout that beset consultation psychiatrists as a result of the many complex problems they routinely face.

The patient population with which the consultation psychiatrist works varies from general medical patients, including those seen in ambulatory settings, to patients seen in more specialized services such as oncology, transplantation surgery, renal dialysis, obstetrics, and gynecology. In each patient population, there are a variety of situations in which consultation psychiatrists will be called. Lipowski (1968) suggested that the various diagnostic problems encountered in consultation psychiatry may be organized in the following fashion.

First, there are those patients whose psychological (i.e., cognitive, behavioral, affective) presentation is the first symptom of an organic disease—the acute and chronic brain syndromes. Consultation psychiatrists must be experts in diagnosing and managing both delirious states and dementing illnesses. Delirium can have various causes, including metabolic derangements attributable to underlying pathophysiological disorders, reactions to a wide variety of medicines, or, as is commonly seen, the acute confusion and disorganization of demented individuals in response to an unfamiliar setting such as the hospital. Next, there are psychological reactions, such as depression and anxiety, to organic disease. Patients may have trouble within the strange and frightening context of a hospital environment or may be reasonably terrified of the implications of a serious illness. Less common are the "psychosomatic disorders" (DSM-IV [American Psychiatric Association 1994] psychological factors affecting medical conditions) such as irritable bowel syndrome or tension headaches. Such disorders are seen by a wide variety of medical practitioners, not just consultation psychiatrists. In addition, consultation psychiatrists often see acute behavioral problems within a medical setting, such as patients with borderline personality disorder who are not complying with medical management or who attempt suicide.

Working with all of these types of patients can present difficult and challenging clinical problems and multiple stresses, and may lead to physician burnout. In addition, it can be distressing to work with medical and nursing staff in emergency care settings who are not always psychologically oriented. To cope with such problems and burnout, it is essential for consultation psychiatrists to develop peer support. There must be cross-coverage to make scheduling easier, the opportunity to discuss different cases to foster intellectual interest, and a strong organizational format within the general medical structure (Wise and Berlin 1981).

Gratification from such work stems from the variety of fascinating and challenging problems a consultation-liaison psychiatrist faces. These psychiatrists can observe the effects of clear stresses upon character structure, and can integrate the biological, psychological, and social aspects into clinical formulations (O'Shanick et al. 1986). Consultation psychiatrists maintain their medical heritage and, on a daily basis, reaffirm a sense of being physicians as well as psychiatrists.

Training Requirements

The Psychiatric Residency Review Committee of the Accreditation Council for Graduate Medical Education requires that residents receive some experience in consultation psychiatry, but in some centers this is a minor part of the total residency program. Thus, it is postresidency fellowships that afford trainees a realistic opportunity to specialize in this field. The Academy of Psychosomatic Medicine has gathered information regarding consultation psychiatry fellowships, but there is no formal certification by the American Board of Medical Specialties or the American Board of Psychiatry and Neurology.

A consultation-liaison fellowship should be busy but provide sufficient time for fellows to read, carry out some research activities, and grow in their identity as psychiatrists. The training experience within a fellowship should consist of certain essential elements (Wise and Brantley 1980). First, clinical experience should be divided between consultation and liaison activities. Both subsets of consultation psychiatry are overlapping and interrelated. These activities should be carefully supervised by faculty; the most efficient means for such supervision is by having regular attending rounds where trainees seeing patients in psychiatric consultation are directly observed by faculty members. Second, trainees' liaison activities with unit staff or specific patients should be supervised, in terms of both reviewing the unique aspects of the liaison area and discussing problems that arise. Such activities should be sufficient to provide a wide variety of clinical experience for the fellow, but should not be of such magnitude that fellows have no time to read or participate in other activities.

Formal didactic experience should include reviewing relevant consultation-liaison literature as well as involvement in other activities of the psychiatry department, such as grand rounds and journal clubs. It is also helpful for consultation-liaison fellows to do outpatient psychotherapy under supervision. This continues to confirm the consultation psychiatrist's identity as a psychiatrist and also helps his or her maturation in this difficult endeavor.

In addition, carefully planned and supervised research is an important part of any fellowship; research seminars that review the basics of research methodology and statistics are essential. Frequently, senior faculty must help develop viable projects that the fellows can carry out. If such expertise is not available, then fellows should be encouraged to develop conferences on case studies of some interesting consultation or liaison subjects. For example, recent research projects at one of our (TNW's) hospitals included the role of depression in alexithymic patients (Wise et al. 1990), compliance with psychiatric consultations by nonpsychiatric physicians (Wise 1987), and a survey of neuroleptic utilization by nonpsychiatric physicians (Wise et al. 1989). It is also important that a fellowship program have adequate resources, including a good medical library and word processing and computer capabilities.

Career Opportunities

Following completion of training, consultation psychiatrists will have a variety of career options. If one wishes to practice consultation psychiatry exclusively, providing consultations and ongoing liaison work, an institutional job is necessary. This can be in a variety of institutional settings, such as a university medical center, a community-based teaching hospital, or a Veterans Administration hospital. Institutional support is important because many consultations are not well reimbursed. First, some patients seen in psychiatric consultation have minimal or no ability to pay for services. However, evaluations for such patients are requested by colleagues, and it is imperative that they be seen, irrespective of their ability to pay. Second, insurance coverage often provides minimal reimbursement for such consultations despite the length of time necessary to carry out a full psychiatric consultation. Finally, liaison psychiatry is rarely financially viable unless the host service is willing to pay; thus, institutional support is essential.

If one wishes to enter private practice, consultation psychiatry is an excellent method of marketing one's abilities. Wise (1987) described the market for consultation psychiatry and remarked that physicians are the consumers of consultation psychiatry. Prompt and effective service is the best advertisement any physician can offer, and consultation psychiatrists can often deliver such service. Effective communication with the consultee is a necessary part of any psychiatric consultation. Thus, although it may be difficult to fund a career in consultation psychiatry outside of an institution, it is wonderful training for general hospital psychiatry careers that are clearly viable private practice options. It may, in fact, be the best training for private practice because it leads the psychiatrist to develop skills in a variety of settings and the ability to work with a group of physicians who will be referral sources in the future.

Legal Challenges

The major legal liability for consultation psychiatrists is with patients who have made suicide attempts or gestures. Thus, consultation psychiatrists must be fully grounded in general psychiatry. The ability to assess individuals with suicidal ideation or history is mandatory.

Psychiatric Liaison with Medical Specialties

Overall, there are increasing numbers of liaison services (i.e., the presence of full- or part-time psychiatrists in other departments) in the United States, though not many in departments of obstetrics and gynecology. There is increasing evidence that these services are cost effective in relation to patient care, days in hospital, and morbidity (Levitan and Kornfeld 1981; Pincus 1984; Rome 1987). Consultation-liaison psychiatry allows for the development of focused careers in specific areas of medicine. As an example, we look at the development of a psychiatric–reproductive biology liaison service.

Liaison With Obstetrics-Gynecology Services

There are exciting prospects for collaboration between psychiatrists and obstetrician-gynecologists (Rosenthal and Smith 1989). The two specialties are growing closer to one another in understanding both biological and psychosocial influences (Good 1972). Specialists in the field of obstetrics and gynecology are facing some of the major biological and social issues of our time (Pasnau 1975), such as acquired immunodeficiency syndrome, abortion, teenage pregnancy, infertility and the possibilities offered by new reproductive technologies, and problems specific to developmental phases such as midlife and menopause. Although labor and delivery have become infinitely safer for mother and infant, there are still high infant mortality rates, a lack of prenatal care, and a malpractice climate that makes physicians in these specialties very concerned.

Liaison psychiatrists practicing within obstetrics-gynecology services must be familiar with all aspects and subtleties applicable to the practice in order to facilitate the interactions and foster mutual respect between themselves and the treating physicians. For example, obstetrician-gynecologists must be at home in a number of settings, from operating and delivery rooms to intensive care units, offices, clinics, and oncology wards. They often must make quick decisions and act immediately, yet also function as educators and counselors. They may love the technological aspects, yet must also understand psychosocial functions (Nadelson and Notman 1977). They are the primary physicians for women of reproductive age and beyond (Nadelson and Notman 1982).

Psychiatrists working closely with obstetricians and gynecologists have a wonderful opportunity for preventive health practice by intervening in situations before they become serious enough to be major mental health problems. For example, they can help in obstetric outpatient clinics by identifying pregnant women who might be at risk for postpartum depression (Appleby et al. 1989) or in infertility clinics by seeing couples who are entering in vitro fertilization programs and discussing with them the stress of these programs and how to diminish it. Patients seen in their own medical settings may experience less stigma connected with a mental health consultation than if they were seen in a psychiatric facility. Also, medical practitioners feel less hostility toward psychiatric colleagues in settings where they work closely together (Small and Mitchell 1979).

An Illustrative Model of Liaison With an Obstetrics-Gynecology Service

Some reproductive biology departments have been willing to support the collaboration between psychiatry and obstetrical-gynecology services in terms of office space, secretarial services, and partial salaries. To illustrate how this might happen, we examine the development of the psychiatric liaison service in the hospital with which one of the authors (MBR) is affiliated, which grew out of a consultation service initially provided by the psychiatry department.

Initially, there were few psychiatric consultations requested by the hospital's obstetrics-gynecology department, and those mainly focused on nurses' concerns that some new mothers leaving the hospital with their newborns might not have the ability to care for a baby. These patients were sent to the psychiatric clinic for consultation but rarely kept their appointments. The other common type of consultation was to write letters for women pursuing abortions.

In 1972, an obstetrics and gynecology liaison service was begun with a psychiatrist and an obstetrician-gynecologist who was also trained in psychiatry. The directors of both departments were very supportive of the liaison. At present, the Division of Behavioral Obstetrics and Gynecology in our hospital has a full-time liaison psychiatrist who works closely with a psychiatric nurse clinician, the nursing staff, social workers, residents, and students in clinical obstetrics and gynecology. Psychiatric residents in their third or fourth year spend about 10 hours a week in the division on 3- to 6-month rotations. A bioethicist with a special interest in women's reproductive health and a research psychologist have also been part of this group.

The curriculum includes a series of seminars for third-year medical students doing their clerkship in reproductive biology (Romano 1964). Topics for these seminars range from normal psychological changes in pregnancy and puerperium to postpartum depression, sexual history taking, psychological aspects of contraception, care of patients who have been raped, the menopausal patient, emotional aspects of gynecological surgery, psychological aspects of infertility and reproductive technologies, and psychological care of oncology patients. In these seminars, students read papers and discuss cases. Many of the same subjects are discussed by staff and residents in both psychiatry and obstetrics and gynecology. Research projects done by residents include a study of women giving up babies for adoption and of panic attacks in pregnancy.

Much clinical education, however, is provided informally in the office, the corridors, the ward, and the labor and delivery suite. There has been a gradual move away from seeing problems as organic or psychological and toward asking which factors and symptoms are biological and which are psychological.

Funding the liaison psychiatrist position has always been a problem, with financing by a combination of fees from patients, third-party payers, a contribution from the medical school for teaching and services for students, and a contribution from the department for general services. Research grants can be helpful as well.

Special Issues in Consultation-Liaison With Obstetrics-Gynecology Services

Consultation-liaison psychiatry is a good field for women, with many role models such as Drs. Grete Bibring, Carol Nadelson, Malkah Notman, Elizabeth Small, Ann Seiden, Roberta Apfel, Donna Stewart, Gail Robinson, and others (Bibring and Valenstein 1976; Rosenthal and Small 1986). Descriptions of their work with obstetrical and gynecological patients have offered much help to those who followed. Many men have also been pioneers in this area—for example, Drs. John Romano, Raphael Good, and Robert Pasnau and his colleagues at the University of California Los Angeles—so obstetrical and gynecological liaison psychiatry is not a field exclusively for women.

The National Institute of Mental Health and the National Institute of Child Health and Human Development have set research into mental health aspects of reproductive function in women over the life cycle as a priority. These organizations hope to see considerably more research in basic sciences related to hormones and brain function; menstrual-related disorders; mood and postpartum psychiatric disorders; issues related to control of reproduction, contraception, and treatment of infertility with the new reproductive technologies; and menopause and mental health. Therefore, young people entering this area have a wonderful opportunity not only for service and teaching, but also for support of their research interests in collaboration with biologists and sociologists.

Conclusion

Consultation-liaison training offers young psychiatrists a broad range of career opportunities in a variety of settings and with a variety of medical specialties. As medicine advances its techniques and capacity to reduce morbidity and mortality, new applications for consultation-liaison work will also develop.

References

American Psychiatric Association: Diagnostic and Statistical Manual of Mental Disorders, 4th Edition. Washington, DC, American Psychiatric Association, 1994

Appleby L, Fox II, Shaw M, et al: The psychiatrist in the obstetric unit. Br J Psychiatry 154:510–515, 1989

Bibring G, Valenstein A: Psychological aspects of pregnancy. Clin Obstet Gynecol 19:357–371, 1976

Brown TM: Descartes, dualism and psychosomatic medicine, in The Anatomy of Madness. Edited by Bynum T, Porter R, Shepherd M. London, Tavistock, 1985, pp 48–62

Good R: The third ear: interviewing techniques in obstetrics and gynecology. Obstet Gynecol 40:760–762, 1972

Hunter R, Macalpine I: Three Hundred Years of Psychiatry. London, Oxford University Press, 1963

Levitan SJ, Kornfeld DS: Clinical and cost benefits of liaison psychiatry. Am J Psychiatry 138:790–793, 1981

Lipowski ZJ: Review of consultation psychiatry and psychosomatic medicine: theoretical issues. Psychosom Med 30:394–422, 1968

Lipowski ZJ: Psychosomatic Medicine and Liaison Psychiatry. New York, Plenum, 1985

McHugh PR, Slavney PR: The Perspectives of Psychiatry. Baltimore, MD, Johns Hopkins University Press, 1983

Meyer E, Mendelson M: Psychiatric consultations with patients on medical and surgical wards: patterns and processes. Psychiatry 24:197–220, 1961

Nadelson C, Notman M: Emotional aspects of the symptoms, functions, and disorders of women, in Psychiatric Medicine. Edited by Usdin G. New York, Brunner/Mazel, 1977, pp 334–397

Nadelson C, Notman M: The Woman Patient, 3 Vols. Vol 1—Sexual and Reproductive Aspects of Women's Health Care; Vol 2—Concepts of Femininity and the Life Cycle; and Vol 3—Aggression, Adaptations and Psychotherapy. New York, Plenum, 1982

O'Shanick GJ, Levenson JL, Wise TN: The general hospital as a center of biopsychosocial training. Gen Hosp Psychiatry 8:365–371, 1986

Pasnau R: Psychiatry and obstetrics and gynecology: report of a 5-year experience in psychiatric liaison, in Consultation-Liaison Psychiatry. Edited by Pasnau R. New York, Grune & Stratton, 1975, pp 135–148

Romano J: Psychosocial aspects of obstetrical-gynecological practice: implications for education, and research. Bulletin of the Sloane Hospital for Women 10:267–274, 1964

Rome J: The marketplace revisited: futures in consultation-liaison psychiatry. Psychiatric Annals 17:79–83, 1987

Rosenthal MB, Small E: Women psychiatrists as consultants to obstetrics and gynecology, in Women Physicians in Leadership Roles. Edited by Dickstein L, Nadelson C. Washington, DC, American Psychiatric Press, 1986, pp 195–204

Rosenthal MB, Smith DH: Liaison psychiatry in obstetrics and gynecology, in The Free Woman: Women's Health in the 1990s. Edited by Van Hall E, Everaerd W. New Jersey, Parthenon Publishing Group, 1989, pp 835–842

Siegel RE: Galen on Psychology, Psychopathology and Function and Diseases of the Nervous System. Basel, Switzerland, Karger, 1973

Small E, Mitchell G: Practical aspects of full-time liaison psychiatry in gynecology. J Reprod Med 22:151–155, 1979

Strain JJ, Grossman S: Psychological Care of the Medically Ill: A Primer in Liaison Psychiatry. New York, Appleton-Century-Crofts, 1974

Weiner H: Psychobiology and Human Disease. New York, Elsevier, 1977

Wise TN: Segmenting and articulating the market in consultation-liaison psychiatry. Gen Hosp Psychiatry 9:354–359, 1987

Wise TN, Berlin R: Burnout: stresses in consultation-liaison psychiatry. Psychosomatics 22:744–751, 1981

Wise TN, Brantley JT: A community hospital based consultation-liaison fellowship: structure and content. Psychosomatics 21:205–212, 1980

Wise TN, Mann LS, Jani N, et al: Haloperidol prescribing practices in the general hospital. Gen Hosp Psychiatry 11:368–374, 1989

Wise TN, Mann LS, Mitchell JD, et al: Secondary alexithymia: an empirical validation. Compr Psychiatry 31:1–6, 1990

Section II: Setting-Related Careers

Outpatient-Based Practice

CHAPTER EIGHT

Private Practice

Kathleen M. Mogul, M.D.
Joseph E. V. Rubin, M.D.

Private practice is a large, vibrant sector of psychiatry accounting for the treatment of a wide spectrum of patients ranging from the troubled to the severely mentally ill. Despite this, many psychiatrists fear that the future of private practice is bleak. Certainly the future characteristics of private practice are unpredictable; changes are taking place and their direction can be guessed, but neither their timing nor their ultimate outcome can be known.

Until recently, psychiatric private practice was almost synonymous with solo practice, and generally included, or mainly consisted of, psychotherapy. Patients paid for services out of pocket, often with reimbursement by private insurers. Psychiatrists had wide latitude regarding treatment modality and duration, but following scientific developments and the amenability of many conditions to treatment with medications, most modified their practices accordingly.

Many recent changes in private practice have followed largely from economic pressures to provide the most efficient treatment at the lowest cost. Changes in private practice that are already discernible and that may become more dominant include the following:

1. A growing tendency to practice in groups, to share increasing overhead costs and diminish isolation
2. Increased hiring by psychiatrists of nonphysician mental health professionals who do psychotherapy or "counseling" at lower cost while the psychiatrists mainly diagnose, supervise, and prescribe medication
3. A trend for psychiatrists to be part of managed care organizations such as health maintenance organizations (HMOs), preferred provider organizations (PPOs), independent practice associations

(IPAs), and so on, and subject to contracts with these—and for patients, in turn, to be limited to obtaining medical services through these organizations
4. Ever-increasing intrusion by government and other payers into choice of modality and treatment duration for both psychiatrists and patients
5. The development of "practice parameters," or treatment standards, by professional specialties, including the American Psychiatric Association (APA) and the American Medical Association (AMA), in order to avoid their imposition by third-party payers or government agencies

Adapting to intrusive requirements of payers presents many difficult choices for psychiatrists and patients. Weighing confidentiality needs against affordability of care is not easy, and mechanisms to reimburse psychiatrists for the amount of time spent communicating with managed care reviewers do not exist.

The institution of some form of universal health insurance is now thought by many health economists to be imminent, and would likely make all reimbursable care subject to some controls over type and length of treatment given.

Throughout medicine, anger at and decreased trust in physicians has led to polarization between physicians (now often called "providers") and patients (now often called "consumers" or "clients") and to increased litigation against physicians, leading, at times, to negative effects on treatment outcome. Psychiatrists, especially private practitioners, remain acutely aware of the overriding importance of individual treatment relationships and of the importance of confidentiality. Private practice affords an opportunity to articulate patients' needs, define and provide the elements of good treatment, and preserve confidentiality; it can be a force in combating the current erosive trends.

Whatever the future holds, we anticipate that a significant number of patients will remain who will want to choose their psychiatrist, have a voice in determining their treatment needs, including intensive psychotherapy, and pay out of pocket, even at financial sacrifice, thus leaving room for psychiatrists to function in some combination of the newer and the more "old-fashioned" private practice models.

Current Data on Practice Patterns

According to a survey of "active" (defined as not in residency or fellowship training and not retired—either APA member or not) psychiatrists conducted by the APA in 1988–1989, 70.8% of these psychiatrists had some private practice, although only 45.1% listed private practice as their primary work setting (as compared with 57.7% in the previous survey, in 1982). Only 38.2% were in *solo* private practice in 1988. The mean number of work settings for a psychiatrist was 2.3, both in 1982 and in 1988–1989. Clearly, private practice is frequently one among these work settings (Dorwart et al. 1992). In 1993, 50% of psychiatrists participated in some form of managed care. This was the lowest participation of any medical specialty (AMA 1993). If figures for psychiatrists parallel those for physicians in general, more young psychiatrists than older psychiatrists are employed.

In 1992, as in other years, psychiatrists (in all settings) had the third lowest mean net annual income ($142,700) among medical specialists, after that of pediatricians and general/family practitioners. Psychiatrists have the lowest practice expenses, lowest mean annual malpractice expenses, and incur the lowest liability claims among all physicians (AMA 1994).

According to a 1991 AMA study, the following were the average and the median (in parentheses) fees for three psychiatric services: psychiatric diagnostic evaluation, $157.20 ($140.00); individual psychotherapy session (50 minutes), $112.70 ($110.00); and family therapy session (50 minutes), $119.20 ($120.00) (AMA 1991).

Characteristics of Private Psychiatric Practice

Private psychiatric practice is much like primary care practice, with patients often making initial contact without physician referral. Psychiatrists often learn details of their patients' lives that were never known by the patients' internist or family physician, not infrequently are the first to recognize signs and symptoms of physical illness, and often help guide and support patients through medical evaluations and treatments. Psychiatrists may remain involved in a person's care for many years, and may be consulted about, or asked to treat, other close family members.

Geographic location affects the character of practice considerably. Psychiatrists practicing in rural or small-town settings may have the most general psychiatric practice, treating patients both in and out of the hospital, encountering the full range of psychiatric diagnoses, and treating patients of all ages. If psychiatric services in the community are limited, psychiatrists may need to treat mainly the sickest patients, using only the most time-efficient methods. In larger urban communities, there may be both opportunities and pressure to have a more specialized practice. Given the trend toward subspecialization, referrals in some locations might depend in part on one's special expertise (e.g., psychopharmacology, geriatric psychiatry).

Depending on interests and expertise, some psychiatrists may have a regularly scheduled office-based practice of ambulatory patients, while others with a special interest in major mental illness may spend considerable time seeing hospitalized patients. Psychiatrists with special expertise may have consultations occupy considerable time.

Advantages of Private Practice

In large part, the advantages of private practice for psychiatrists coincide with the advantages for their patients. They can choose to work with each other on the basis of compatibility, convenience, fee, and mutually agreed-upon treatment plans. Patients looking for psychotherapy often talk with several clinicians (including non-psychiatrists) before making a choice, a process stressful to both but one that allows for questions and misgivings to be dealt with before a treatment decision. The psychiatrist's medical education and psychopharmacological expertise are often an advantage, but there are patients who are scared off by this, unless psychiatrists can reassure them that medication is not the only option and that their own wishes will be respected.

Patients and physicians in private practice can together address treatment plans and duration as well as fees to be within the patients' means. After termination of treatment, patients can return, as needed, and have the opportunity to be followed over many years. Experienced practitioners know that a consistent, stable treatment relationship and reliable availability, including during crises, lead to fewer extraordinary demands and may, at times, prevent hospitalization.

Private practice may offer particular advantages to women—and an increasing number of men—during those years when they may choose to schedule work somewhat around their families' needs. It is easier to reduce or increase work hours by small increments in private practice than it is in most salaried jobs.

Thus, private practice offers a number of freedoms: choice of work setting and work hours, selection of those patients the psychiatrist feels best able to treat, and the flexibility to recommend treatment modalities and length of treatment with maximum attention to quality of care. Another prominent advantage of private practice is the satisfaction derived from one-to-one interaction with patients.

Drawbacks of Private Practice

Work hours can, of course, be set only within certain limits: appointment hours in the early morning or evening and on Saturday for patients who hold jobs are commonly needed, with extra times—day or night—for patients in crisis. Furthermore, the dependence of patients on their psychiatrists and on an accustomed schedule makes spontaneity and sudden changes in personal plans by the psychiatrist almost impossible, a limitation that can at times be experienced as very restrictive. Thus, vacations and other absences need to be planned well in advance and appropriate coverage arranged.

Psychiatrists in private practice have to accept and cope with some of the inevitable isolation stemming from the many hours spent behind closed doors in one-on-one work with patients, often listening relatively passively rather than "doing." Unless a physician's emotional needs are met by family, friends, collegial exchange and support, and good coping mechanisms, this isolation can lead to distress and physical or emotional symptoms and may eventually contribute to idiosyncratic therapeutic ideas and practices, to dysfunctional and unethical acts such as substance abuse, and even to inappropriate business, personal, and sexual involvements with patients.

Without the frequent casual case-oriented consultations available to many physicians, psychiatrists in private practice must schedule time, often at their own cost and inconvenience, for meetings with colleagues or for supervision. To do this is vitally important to mitigate the negative consequences of professional isolation.

Burnout for the private practitioner may be attributable less to total work demands than to an excessive responsibility borne alone and to a lack of diversity of work. Paradoxically, the remedy may be for the psychiatrist to add involvements, as in a variety of educational and other professional activities, which bring their own different responsibilities and demands. Other means of achieving diversification and acquiring collegial interaction and informal peer consultation are to spend one day each week practicing in a community mental health center or consulting to a variety of community agencies. Scheduled peer consultation groups and purchased individual case supervision help to guard against overlooking treatment approaches and problems as well as allow the private practice psychiatrist to share treatment responsibility.

More mundane disadvantages have to do, in various ways, with the fact that a private practice is in effect a small business for which the psychiatrist has full responsibility, financial and otherwise. Retirement planning has to be considered early, as well as other needs (health, disability, liability, and malpractice insurance) that are parts of benefit packages provided psychiatrists in other settings. Continued referrals need to be encouraged. In addition to the usual clinical and financial record keeping, psychiatrists must now deal with multiple third parties, their requests for documentation and information, and their ever-changing and differing forms.

Practitioners and patients alike must often endure intrusions of treatment reviews by managed care companies and insurers, and HMO stipulations, such as requirements for referral from a "gatekeeper" physician. These types of insurers sometimes require frequent reports and detailed personal information on patients in order to authorize reimbursements. Private practitioners are in the best position to discuss these matters with their patients and to come to reasonable, collaborative decisions to safeguard patients' privacy and best interests.

The additional secretarial help needed to keep up with these administrative tasks, formerly accomplished quickly and easily, adds complexity and expense to a practice and diminishes patient confidentiality, as does increased computerization of insurance and billing data. In the current more regulated and litigious climate, practitioners need to pay special attention to proper clinical documentation and to regulations and laws affecting practice.

How to Start in Private Practice

Many training programs now address the difficult transition from relatively sheltered residency to the more independent career paths that follow. Private practice is the most independent of these, and causes anxiety for most young psychiatrists. Training programs can provide discussion sessions, opportunities for advice from experienced practitioners and from those who made this transition more recently, and other formats for nitty-gritty "how to" questions. It can be extremely valuable for a resident to identify a current or former supervisor in private practice as a mentor or role model to help him or her get started (Borus 1978).

Geographic location. One of the first practical decisions a new private practice psychiatrist must make is the geographic location in which to establish a practice. Sometimes the path of least resistance is to stay in the location of one's training. A resident may have seen a few private patients toward the end of training and anticipate ready-made referral sources in former teachers and peers. Frequently, however, training centers are particularly saturated with private psychiatric services, and anticipated referrals may not materialize.

Lifestyle considerations include whether one wants to live and work in a city, suburb, or rural location. What do these offer as work settings and as places to live, perhaps raise a family, and spend leisure time? In small communities, encounters with patients or their families outside the treatment setting and acquaintances among patients are more common, and the effect on the psychiatrist's practice and personal life needs to be considered. In such settings, coverage arrangements also may require added effort, and continued education may be more difficult.

Patient population. A psychiatrist starting out in private practice should determine what type of patient population he or she wants to serve. After choosing possible settings, the community's need for another psychiatrist should be assessed. Are there special populations that need services, such as children, elderly persons, or underserved and underprivileged populations? Are there large populations of non-native cultures or those whose primary language is not English? Minority populations might be a special magnet for some minority psychiatrists, whereas others may need to assess opportunities and acceptance in communities without such populations.

Office setting. In choosing an office, beginning practitioners often start by subletting or sharing office space. Later they may have to decide between an office in their home or one in a medical or general office building. A home office has both advantages and disadvantages to consider: it saves rental expenses, may offer tax savings, and avoids commuting time and annoyance from early morning or late-day cancellations. Parking is easy and free, but public transportation for patients may not be available. In addition, in small communities, an in-home office may not give patients the anonymous feeling they can achieve in office buildings. Psychiatrists with an in-home practice must be more selective in choosing their patients in order to avoid risking behavior that could be intrusive, or even dangerous, to themselves, family, and neighbors. Furthermore, practice in a home office may make it harder to leave work behind at the end of the workday.

All psychiatric offices must offer good arrangements for soundproofing to protect patients' confidentiality and to keep out noise. This may require costly expert consultation and construction. Especially in communities where patients may know each other, offices and waiting areas with entrances and exits arranged to prevent encounters between successive patients may be necessary.

Combinations of private and institutional practice. Will private practice be part-time or full-time? Because it takes time to build up a patient load and stable cash flow, a young psychiatrist may wish to work at an agency or hospital part-time as an adjunct to a beginning private practice. A well-chosen job is also a way to meet other professionals in a new community, leading to personal rewards and possible referrals. Even later, a part-time job provides variety and protection against the isolation of private practice (see above). It may also be an opportunity to collaborate with other mental health professionals and may provide a satisfying sense of public service if severely ill, needy, or homeless patients are served.

Working with managed care plans. Increasingly, psychiatrists in private practice choose to become members of managed care plans—HMOs, PPOs, IPAs—to increase their referrals. Prior to deciding to join such plans, psychiatrists should consider the legal, financial, and ethical risks associated with participation in each plan and obtain legal consultation before any contract is signed.

Working with other mental health professionals. Similar considerations apply to any psychiatrist deciding to practice with or employ other mental health professionals or to provide medication coverage to patients who have other primary therapists. These arrangements open up avenues toward having more patients and greater income, but treatment complications can result that may require considerable time and communication to remedy as well as pose ethical or legal risks.

Building up a practice. Marketing one's practice requires attention both when starting a practice and as an ongoing necessity. Advertising is now ethically permissible, although deception in advertising or the promising of guaranteed results is not. Appropriate and desirable marketing can lead a psychiatrist to become well established and valued in a community.

It is often advantageous for a private practice psychiatrist to become a member of the active staff of one or more community hospitals, which generally includes obligations to assume care of some hospitalized patients, provide a part of evening and weekend coverage, and consult for other staff physicians. This allows the beginning psychiatrist's clinical ability to be recognized, provides needed continuing medical education opportunities, and allows for less formal case consultation.

If a new psychiatrist has an area of special expertise otherwise lacking in the community, this is a magnet for particular referrals. Prompt response to referrals with rapid, useful feedback to referring physicians and willingness, initially, to treat patients at reduced fees will also encourage referrals.

Another means of becoming established in a new community is to do volunteer work in areas in which the community has a need, which will create publicity and goodwill for the psychiatrist. The community's needs could also suggest topics for lectures or discussion groups held in the community through the school system, clubs, religious groups, or patient advocacy organizations.

Membership in professional organizations. Membership in professional psychiatric and medical societies, including the American Medical Women's Association (AMWA), makes for important contacts and networks within one's professional community.

All these professional and community involvements also provide supports and personal pleasures and a very emotionally rewarding sense of service.

Finally, psychiatrists must initiate and maintain coverage relationships with colleagues. This can be a surprisingly complex task on which may hinge the survival of a practice, particularly in a small community. Availability and communication of mutual expectations must be very clear.

Supports

We cannot overemphasize the need for supports. The psychiatrist in private practice is more subject to the stresses and risks of the "workaholic" physician than other physicians. To derive an excessive amount of one's life satisfaction from work places a burden hazardous to treatment on the intrinsically intense relationship with a relatively small number of patients.

Thus, it is essential that psychiatrists provide for a reasonably satisfying outside life. Despite anxieties about building and maintaining an adequate caseload, a limit on work hours should be planned and followed. Ample leisure and vacation time must be scheduled. At times of illness, private practitioners should recognize when self-care demands an interruption of work rather than giving in to the inclination to "tough it out."

Various needs for help should be recognized. Clerical and accounting help, and often, particularly for women, household help are among the more mundane aspects of not trying to "do it all." Continued case supervision or consultation, when needed, from a respected colleague concerning difficult patients offers continued learning and help around treatment problems and even legal protection with complaints or lawsuits that may arise later. Psychiatrists should also be alert to those times when stresses of work or personal life threaten to be overwhelming and they themselves would benefit from professional help. The difficulty in obtaining this should not be made into an obstacle to receiving needed help.

Conclusion

In private practice, individual work with patients is often demanding and lonely, at times seeming interminable; sometimes it seems that family members, insurers, health planners, government agencies, and indeed the whole spectrum of social contexts within which practitioner and patient meet are conspiring to undermine both treatment and professional satisfaction. Yet private practice persists despite predictions over a decade ago of its imminent demise; this survival is attributable in large part to the fact that rewards for patients and psychiatrists alike are often as gratifying as the obstacles are great.

References

American Medical Association: Physician Marketplace Statistics. Chicago, IL, AMA, 1991

American Medical Association: Physician Characteristics and Distribution in the United States. Chicago, IL, AMA, 1993

American Medical Association: Socioeconomic Characteristics of Medical Practice. Chicago, IL, AMA, 1994

Borus JF: The transition to practice seminar. Am J Psychiatry 135:1513–1516, 1978

Dorwart RA, Chartock LR, Dial T, et al: A national study of psychiatrists' professional activities. Am J Psychiatry 149:11, 1499–1505, 1992

For Further Reading

Bittker TE: The industrialization of American psychiatry. Am J Psychiatry 142:149–154, 1985

Logsdon L: Establishing a Private Psychiatric Practice. Washington, DC, American Psychiatric Press, 1985

The business of psychiatry. Psychiatric Annals (special issue) 14:316–392, 1984

CHAPTER NINE

Psychiatric Practice in Industry

David B. Robbins, M.D., M.P.H.

Introduction

Occupational psychiatry is an informal subspecialty—an area of specialized practice that has not been formally accredited and that does not have prescribed training or specialty certification—integrating information and concepts derived from several social science and medical disciplines. Relevant social sciences include anthropology, sociology, economics, management, social psychology, and organizational development. Although a psychiatric subspecialty, occupational psychiatry is closely related to occupational medicine, physiology, addiction research, military psychiatry, school psychiatry, penal psychiatry, and forensic medicine (Robbins 1986). The principal locus of intervention is the interface between individual psychodynamics and the system dynamics of the work organization (Giannandrea 1985; Robbins 1986; Rohrlich 1980). A psychiatrist who practices in a social system characterized by significant work roles (e.g., schools, prisons, military services, private or public industry) focuses on the fit between the individual and the work roles prescribed by the organization (McLean 1970). This unique interdisciplinary focus, the essence of occupational psychiatry, is exemplified by the following case history.

> Ms. E, a 33-year-old married administrative specialist, was referred for psychiatric consultation because of "work stress." Her complaints included interrupted sleep, tachycardia with palpitations, and binge eating. A compulsively compliant woman who always attempted to please people, Ms. E could not refuse demands, even if they made her work load excessive. Her long hours of overtime were aggravated by her installing a computer terminal in her home, thereby weakening the boundary between workplace and family. She supported an aggressive, ambitious marketing group; most of the managers had little time for, nor interest

in, the administrative aspects of their work and were more than willing to delegate these tasks to Ms. E. Psychiatric consultation focused on the interplay between the expanding demands of the work group and the conscience-supported immaturities of this compulsive person. With the help of her own psychotherapist, Ms. E was able to restore a balance in her life, allocate time for personal needs and family, and set appropriate limits at work.

Although germinal elements of occupational psychiatry are found in the medical writings of antiquity, the field developed a specific identity during and after World War I (American Psychiatric Association 1984). Giberson, engaged by Metropolitan Life Insurance Company in 1922, was the first full-time psychiatrist in American industry. Anderson published the first textbook on occupational psychiatry in 1929 (American Psychiatric Association 1984). Other major texts were those written by Ross (1956) and Collins (1961). During World War II, occupational psychiatry contributed to the maintenance of mental health for both military and civilian populations.

The field grew larger and more sophisticated in the four postwar decades. The American Psychiatric Association's (APA's) Committee on Occupational Psychiatry published "Troubled People on the Job" in 1959 and "The Mentally Ill Employee" in 1965. The burgeoning literature was compiled and abstracted by the National Clearinghouse for Mental Health Information from 1965 to 1970 and by the Cornell University Center for Occupational Mental Health from 1971 to 1973 (American Psychiatric Association 1984).

In 1982, the profound community mental health effects of job loss, precipitated by corporate plant closings, mergers and acquisitions, staff reductions, and other factors, were examined by the Group for the Advancement of Psychiatry's (GAP's) Committee on Psychiatry in Industry. Their 1982 monograph, "Job Loss—A Psychiatric Perspective," clearly integrated national and local economic events with individual mental health, including self-esteem, family functioning, work capacity, and suicide. The following two case examples illustrate the significance of work in maintaining self-esteem:

> Mr. F, a 55-year-old married man with one son, had worked for the same company for 35 years. He had few avocational interests, relying on his job to provide emotional support and meaning in his life. During a national recession, his company decided to close Mr. F's branch, thereby eliminating his job.

Despite an offer to fill a similar post with the company in another city, Mr. F became depressed and suicidal.

Mr. G, a long-term employee of a large technical manufacturing and marketing company, successfully coped with a series of midlife losses and disappointments. These included his children's departure for college, his wife's increasing dependence on alcohol, and his father's progressive enfeeblement. However, when his department, which had been developed for years with his guidance, was phased out because of changing business needs, Mr. G became asthmatic and depressed.

At the present time, at least 130 psychiatrists participate in occupational psychiatry full- or part-time (American Academy of Organizational and Occupational Psychiatry 1994). Three organizations support occupational psychiatry, providing collegial exchange of information and ideas: GAP's Committee on Psychiatry in Industry, APA's Committee on Occupational Psychiatry, and the American Academy of Organizational and Occupational Psychiatry (AAOP).

Current Positions in Occupational Psychiatry

At present, occupational psychiatrists hold positions as consultants, teachers, writers, and researchers. In most instances, they have played a major part in creating their specific jobs. Perhaps to a greater degree than other psychiatric subspecialties, occupational psychiatry requires an entrepreneurial spirit. For example, one contemporary occupational psychiatrist started a firm that provides developmental evaluation, organizational consultation, and employee assistance programs (EAPs). Another colleague designed and implemented a leadership research and training institute.

Research and Teaching

Research and teaching currently focus on specific clinical problems encountered in industry (e.g., psychiatric injury); issues related to sexual discrimination and harassment of women in the workplace (Bursten 1986); difficulties created by loss of work through mergers, layoffs, acquisitions, and so on (Group for the Advancement of Psychiatry 1982); work stress (McLean 1970); and problems of troubled executives (Speller 1989). Although some of this work takes place in medical school psychiatry departments, most of the recent contributions have been generated in departments of public health, preventive medicine, or occupational medicine or in independent occupational medicine-psychiatry clinics (e.g., The Center of Occupational Psychiatry in San Francisco, California) (Brodsky 1988; Enelow 1988; Larsen 1988).

As evidenced by the size and diversity of the occupational psychiatry literature, many practitioners publish their ideas and observations. Much of this work appears in business and industrial psychology journals (e.g., human resources management articles in *The Harvard Business School Review,* articles on psychiatry in industry in *Fortune,* articles on family life issues in the *Bank Street School Newsletter*) rather than in traditional psychiatric sources. Because occupational psychiatrists function in a diversity of positions, their writings cover a wide range of interventions, from individual psychotherapy (Rohrlich 1980; Speller 1989) to corporate or national policy determinations (Group for the Advancement of Psychiatry 1982; London et al. 1988). London et al.'s (1988) collaboration with Commissioner Loeb regarding workers' compensation and psychiatric liability exemplifies psychiatric consultation in strategic decisions. The intended audience of these writings varies considerably: Carone (1982) and Robbins (1988) addressed occupational physicians; American Psychiatric Association (1985), Brodsky (1988), Giannandrea (1985), Larsen (1988), and Rigaud (1989) addressed psychiatrists; American Psychiatric Association (1965), McLean (1970), Robbins (1986), and Speller (1989) addressed managers and personnel specialists; and Rohrlich (1980) addressed general readers.

Consultation

The center of occupational psychiatry practice is consultation (American Psychiatric Association 1984; Rigaud 1989; Robbins 1986), but this type of psychiatric consultation is not limited to traditional clinical practice, which usually involves one patient and a treating or examining physician. In occupational psychiatry, consultation may involve system interventions at different levels, from the specific individual, to small work groups, to entire corporate organizations. Frequently, consultations assist in balancing individual patient-employee needs with the well-being of the entire enterprise (McLean 1970). Take the following as examples:

- A midwestern practitioner created seminars for senior managers and administrators. With his guidance, clients were able to share the difficulties of managing at the highest levels of responsibility.
- With a solid academic base, a New England psychiatrist aided companies in diminishing the stress of plant closings, staff reductions, and acquisition-mergers.

Psychiatrists who provide advice and counsel to senior management have previously learned the intricacies of corporate culture by consulting at lower levels of the organization or by studying pertinent subjects in graduate schools of business or public health. For example, one psychiatric entrepreneur holds an M.B.A. and a psychoanalytic certificate. Another colleague began his consultation experience with traditional individual evaluations. As his reputation grew within the organization, he was asked to assist with policy determinations. He then gained additional expertise by returning to graduate school for an M.P.H. Unlike consultation in a health care facility, occupational psychiatry requires interactions with managers, lawyers, personnel specialists, and administrators.

Consultants continue to develop clear ethical guidelines for their practice (American Psychiatric Association 1985; Larsen 1988).

Future Opportunities

The essential activities of occupational psychiatry—research, teaching, writing, and consulting—will continue to provide opportunities in the next decade. But the structure of service provision will, by necessity, evolve as corporate organizations cope with changing economic conditions. Successful practice will require a capacity to accurately measure emerging conditions and to adapt rapidly to them. For example, many support services previously supplied to corporations by in-house professionals will be provided by external "vendors." This trend is already apparent in occupational medicine, including psychiatry. Vendors may be individual consultants (currently the dominant model) or aggregate organizations developed to provide diverse services to business firms with various needs (Larsen 1988).

Employee Assistance Programs

As the employee assistance movement matures, psychiatrists may become more involved in these programs, principally as designers and supervisors of the programs (American Psychiatric Association 1989; Brill et al. 1985). For thousands of work organizations, EAPs serve as gatekeepers for all mental health problems and benefits. Most of the EAPs were started by substance abuse counselors and psychologists. Few programs had any psychiatric involvement and few referred workers to psychiatrists except for emergencies. The EAPs headed by psychiatrists have gradually gained increasing acceptance based on the thoroughness of their evaluations and their ability to manage complex clinical situations. The 1990s are seeing an expanding role for occupational psychiatrists in EAPs.

Health Care Management

Health care management, including management of benefits and disability programs, represents a growing industry in which psychiatrists should play a major part. Some psychiatrists are already employed as executives in insurance companies, with responsibility for controlling mental health benefits. Health care management will include disability determination, investigation of alternative treatment schemata, and design of flexible benefit packages for industry. Some jobs will involve traditional clinical evaluation and treatment prescription; others will demand administrative and consulting skills. These changes will parallel developments in the community (e.g., more counseling and psychotherapy may be provided by nonmedical therapists; psychiatrists may spend more of their time evaluating patients for medications, supervising the work of counselors, and consulting with other physicians).

Coping With Current Business Trends

Finally, American business will have an increasing need for psychiatric advice to cope with changes in the work environment if that advice is truly informed. International competition and a global marketplace coupled with important demographic changes in the American workforce (e.g., increasing numbers of women and minorities) require structural and procedural changes with increasing velocity.

Inevitably, work stress will increase (McLean 1970). Industry will seek help in buffering employees from adverse effects of stress. Employees' ability to successfully cope with all these changes will be a major determinant of corporate profitability (Speller 1989). Psychiatrists can and should assist senior management in adopting policies that facilitate change with a minimum of distress. Specific areas in which occupational psychiatrists can have positive impact include accurate and timely communication about change, assistance with job search and placement, provision of critical benefits during transitions, and provision of social support, including counseling. Company leaders must also give clear indications of concern about the effects of change on the workforce.

Conclusions and Recommendations

It will be increasingly rare for privately practicing psychiatrists to devote all of their time to direct patient care. To prepare adequately for other activities, new skills and attitudes must be acquired. One important change must be a shift in focus from unidimensional intervention to a general systems approach, with particular attention to interface issues involving the individual and the organization. Psychiatrists may have to surrender some of their autonomy (e.g., private office practice) in exchange for participation in complex work groups. They may need to move from positions of direct care provision to roles as teachers and advisers. Therefore, residents and beginning practitioners require experience in consultation-liaison service, teaching, and administration to ready themselves for opportunities in occupational psychiatry.

Formal training programs in occupational psychiatry have appeared periodically and should be developed anew during this last decade of the 20th century (American Psychiatric Association 1984). Such programs could be joint efforts of psychiatry departments and graduate faculties of occupational medicine or business. A model curriculum would include review of relevant social science literature, with emphasis on general systems theory; review of occupational medicine; supervised clinical experience in private industry or government workplaces; seminars with policy makers, including business executives, labor union leaders, and government officials; teaching experiences in both medical and nonmedical settings (e.g., stress seminars for business, disability process discussion groups for physicians); and research and publication, with emphasis on problems considered critical by industry (e.g., absenteeism, morale and productivity, leadership, equal opportunity versus discrimination, substance abuse rehabilitation).

Until residency and fellowship programs are established, physicians interested in occupational psychiatry should begin by perusing the extensive literature on occupational medicine, including psychiatry, business, personnel, and industrial psychology. They should pay particular attention to concepts of system levels and integration, read articles by senior managers expressing their concerns for the future, consider how they could use their expertise in interpersonal relations to help management, and seek the advice and counsel of experienced consultants. Finally, they should not wait in their private offices for opportunity to knock. They should develop programs and the entrepreneurial spirit to successfully sell them!

References

American Academy of Organizational and Occupational Psychiatry: Membership Directory. Dallas, TX, AAOP, 1994

American Psychiatric Association, Committee on Abuse and Misuse of Psychiatry in the United States: Position statement on employment-related psychiatric examinations. Am J Psychiatry 142:416, 1985

American Psychiatric Association, Committee on Occupational Psychiatry: Troubled People on the Job. Washington, DC, APA, 1959

American Psychiatric Association, Committee on Occupational Psychiatry: The Mentally Ill Employee, His Treatment and Rehabilitation—A Guide for Management. New York, Harper & Row, 1965

American Psychiatric Association, Committee on Occupational Psychiatry: Employee assistance programs and the role of the psychiatrist: report of the Committee on Occupational Psychiatry. Am J Psychiatry 146:690–694, 1989

American Psychiatric Association, Task Force on Psychiatry and Industry: Report of the Task Force on Psychiatry and Industry. Am J Psychiatry 9:1139–1144, 1984

Anderson VV: Psychiatry in Industry. New York, Harper & Brothers, 1929

Brill P, Herzberg J, Speller J: Employee assistance programs: an overview and suggested roles for psychiatrists. Hosp Community Psychiatry 36:727–732, 1985

Brodsky C: The psychiatry epidemic in the American workplace. Occupational Medicine: State of the Art Reviews 3:653–662, 1988

Bursten B: Psychiatric injury in women's workplaces. Bull Am Acad Psychiatry Law 14:245–251, 1986

Carone P: History of Mental Health in Industry: The Last Hundred Years. New York, Human Sciences Press, 1982

Collins R: A Manual of Neurology and Psychiatry in Occupational Medicine. New York, Grune & Stratton, 1961

Enelow A: Assessing the effect of psychiatric disorders on work function. Occupational Medicine: State of the Art Reviews 3:621–627, 1988

Giannandrea P: Psychodynamic approach to occupational psychiatry: comparative case studies and review. Am J Psychother 39:421–430, 1985

Group for the Advancement of Psychiatry, Committee on Psychiatry in Industry: Job Loss—A Psychiatric Perspective. New York, Mental Health Materials Center, 1982

Larsen R: Ethical issues in psychiatry and occupational medicine. Occupational Medicine: State of the Art Reviews 3:719–726, 1988

London D, Zonana H, Loeb R: Workers compensation and psychiatric disability. Occupational Medicine: State of the Art Reviews 3:595–609, 1988

McLean A: Mental Health and Work Organizations. Chicago, IL, Rand McNally, 1970

Rigaud M: A model of consultation in occupational psychiatry. Hosp Community Psychiatry 40:745–747, 1989

Robbins D: The psychiatric patient at work. Occupational Medicine: State of the Art Reviews 1:549–557, 1986

Robbins D: Psychiatric conditions in worker fitness and risk evaluation. Occupational Medicine: State of the Art Reviews 3:309–321, 1988

Rohrlich J: Work and Love: The Crucial Balance. New York, Summit Books, 1980

Ross W: Practical Psychiatry for Industrial Physicians. Springfield, IL, Charles C Thomas 1956

Speller J: Executives in Crisis. San Francisco, CA, Jossey-Bass, 1989

CHAPTER TEN

Psychiatric Practice in College and University Mental Health Services

Leah J. Dickstein, M.D.

Historical Development

During the first two decades of the 20th century, a small group of psychiatrists began working in the area of *educational psychiatry*—that is, providing psychiatric services on college campuses to troubled students (Blain 1968). Dana L. Farnsworth, M.D., Henry K. Oliver Professor of Hygiene and Director of University Health Services at Harvard University, clearly recognized as one of the founders and earliest authors in the field of college mental health, served for almost four decades at Harvard and two other institutions. He identified the field's pioneers:

> Stewart Paton at Princeton (1910), Smiley Blanton at the University of Wisconsin (1914), Karl Menninger at Washburne College, Kansas (1920), H. M. Kearns, full-time psychiatrist at the United States Military Academy at West Point (1920), Arthur Ruggles at Dartmouth and Yale (1921, 1925), and Austen Fox Riggs at Vassar (1923) were among the first psychiatrists to appreciate the possibilities for prevention of crippling emotional conflict among students by working on causes of distress with both students and faculty members rather than waiting for the classic syndromes of illness to appear. (Farnsworth 1966, p. 3)

Above all else a humane physician and therefore also an educator, Farnsworth, along with his early colleagues, realized that psychiatrists' roles on college and university campuses entailed additional roles as educators to the college community at large (Glasscote and Fishman 1973). These pioneering psychiatrists recognized that administrators and faculty could sometimes assist students in understanding and resolving personal developmental crises if the former were aware of warning signs. Thus, generally on a part-time basis, early college psychiatrists assumed responsibility for educating their colleagues about problems students might be burdened with, and about normal and problematic adolescent and young adult personal development (Whittington 1963).

Problems Encountered at Student Mental Health Services

Who are the students who seek professional help from student health service psychiatrists? In 1966, Farnsworth, in his classic text *Psychiatry, Education, and the Young Adult,* detailed the then-current college psychiatric population as follows:

> 10% of students will have emotional conflicts of sufficient severity to warrant professional help, 3% to 4% will have feelings of depression severe enough to impair their efficiency, 1% to 2% will be apathetic and unable to organize their efforts, 2% to 5% will be so adversely affected by past family experiences that they will be unable to control their impulses (character disorders), 5 to 20 students per 10,000 will attempt suicide and 1 to 3 will succeed, [and] 15 to 25 students will become ill enough to require treatment in a mental hospital. (Farnsworth 1966, p. 6)

Farnsworth also stated unequivocally that even academically superior students were vulnerable to becoming psychiatric patients and, most importantly, that most student problems originated prior to college entrance rather than as a consequence of excessive academic pressures. Although most would agree that the percentage of depressed and suicidal students has increased in the past three decades, and that students bring other problems to college psychiatrists that were unrecognized in earlier decades, the fundamental belief remains correct—that is, most personal problems that propel students to seek psychiatric care on campus are, in fact, not acute but had developed much earlier, remained unsolved, and therefore accompanied students to college.

Common problems. Students' chief complaints and psychiatric histories can include all degrees of loss—by death, abandonment, or rejection; all degrees of violence from within and outside the home; all degrees of depression; increasing numbers of anxiety disorders, including panic, phobic, and obsessive-compulsive disorders; and rare psychotic and bipolar disorders. At times, half to two-thirds of the students' histories include alcoholism in their three-generational family histories and, within themselves, any and all of the other addictions. Eating disorders of all types and causes, and even shoplifting, are common chief complaints. Incest; recent date or gang rape; remote history of rape, pregnancy, abortion, children given up for adoption, or personal adoption; problems with heterosexual and homosexual relationships; spousal abuse; child abuse; and sexual identity crises are frequent problems. Other sensitive issues that students either present directly or discuss in response to empathic questioning include acknowledging one's being gay, lesbian, or bisexual, and deciding whether to share this with one's family; deciding to deal with the remote loss of biological and adoptive parents; and dealing with one's own divorce, relationship breakups, and rejection experiences.

Students may have problems with their own children and may need parent counseling or referral. Other student problems may be those of the physically handicapped and chronically ill. Increasingly, chief complaints relate to minority issues, including racism, religious discrimination, and sexism, and to posttraumatic stress disorder of returning veterans and of abuse victims.

Relationship problems. Despite the first men's movement of the 1970s, which followed the second women's movement of the 1960s, I have noted current relationship rejections to be of particular importance to young men, who do not easily recognize, accept, and work through their usually denied vulnerable and dependent feelings (Dickstein 1986). This general lack of ability to resolve feelings of rejection and to accept feelings of helplessness, dependency, and emotional pain lead too many young undergraduate and graduate men to threaten, attempt, or complete suicides, or to become severely depressed or resort to acting out in other violent ways. For both women and men, unresolved issues surrounding remote and recent losses are very common, painful, and clearly important. Losses of parents by death, divorce, separation, and disappearance leave scars that must be worked through. Young adults from divorced families may have experienced several parental divorces, not simply one; often, parental physical, sexual, and emotional abuse occurred in the context of stepparent relationships or was sustained from unofficial parental figures.

College psychiatrists must be well informed about the new psychology of women and men so they can recognize related issues in their student patients, even when the students may not recognize this factor. Often, single-sex group therapy experiences for young adults and for older students, as well as survivors' groups, eating disorders groups, and adult children of alcoholic groups, prove invaluable in helping students reach a more mature understanding of themselves and their problems, and implement constructive solutions. They also experience trust and group support, often for the first time in their lives.

Suicidality. Evaluating suicidal potential is clearly the most difficult responsibility of a college psychiatrist, especially as the suicide rate for adolescents has risen astronomically in the last 25 years. My recent, unpublished data from a 14-year review of suicides among 18-year-old to 28-year-old individuals in one urban county revealed that the rate for completed suicides among women is approaching that of men. These factors highlight the need for college psychiatrists to be constantly attuned to this potential in all of their student patients. Equally important is the responsibility to educate university personnel and other health and mental health professionals about this major issue.

Student diversity. Student diversity is another challenge and opportunity to be met. Part-time students (who often work full-time), international students, and increasing numbers of minority and handicapped students seek or are mandated to seek psychiatric services because of symptomatic dysfunction.

Roles of the Student Health Psychiatrist

Direct Service—Evaluation and Treatment Services

Mental health service sites obviously vary for each school; often they are in separate buildings from classrooms and administrative offices. Available college services also vary greatly. Junior colleges usually employ nurse health service directors and nonpsychiatric mental health professionals. Some four-year institutions, particularly those with graduate and professional schools, usually employ at least one part-time psychiatric consultant who may spend the remainder of the work week in private practice or in a university's department of psychiatry.

Other mental health services are usually staffed by a variety of mental health professionals: one to several psychiatrists working full- or part-time, clinical and counseling psychologists, and social workers; more recently, alcohol education specialists and art therapists have been added. In addition, chaplain trainees and trainees in all mental health disciplines may rotate for several months to a year under supervision. Most mental health service professionals work well with psychiatric consultants in settings of mutual professional respect and concern for patients' appropriate care (Talley and Rockwell 1985).

Services offered are usually short-term, lasting for 6–10 visits, though many schools attempt to provide group experiences for one to two semesters. Brief therapy, cognitive and behavioral therapy, support and therapy groups, relaxation exercises, expressive therapies, and combinations of these can clearly assist impaired students.

Consultation Services

College psychiatrists, whether full- or part-time administrators or consultants, can play a major role in meeting with advisers; faculty; administrators; academic, dormitory, and special services counselors; and public safety officers on a proactive, scheduled basis. These opportunities should be developed and used as a chance to exchange information and as an educational experience for the myriad of university employees who are in contact with more students, and therefore more students with problems, than psychiatrists can ever be.

A system for emergency and nonemergency consultations must be established. In addition, psychiatrists should describe common issues, problems, signs, and symptoms, and encourage interested staff to question students if staff concerns are aroused. Staff will then know whom to contact and which agencies are available for referral.

Because of the increasing numbers of older first- and second-career students on campus today, campus staff should know about community agencies for children, as well as couple and family therapy opportunities.

Supervision of Trainees

Rotations at college mental health or counseling services are usually eagerly sought electives by fourth-year residents or fellows. Generally, these are for 6- to 12-month periods, either full-time or, more commonly, part-time with concomitant supervision. Residents generally enjoy the challenge and opportunity to interact with students who appear so like themselves and often present problems similar to those residents may have had or may not yet have worked through. At other times, residents' education is enhanced by working with international students or with those from other ethnic groups or geographic backgrounds.

Transference and countertransference issues must be raised and resolved appropriately in supervision. A trainee's proximity in age, education, and culture to student-patients often increases the degree of transference and countertransference encountered. Ethical issues of social and sexual exploitation of this patient population must be discussed proactively.

Special Considerations in College Psychiatry

Confidentiality. Clearly, a primary and major concern for student-patients as well as for psychiatrists is maintenance of confidentiality. This is not an easy task in the environs of a close-knit community such as a college, even for those who live off campus. Psychiatrists and all those who refer students for evaluation and treatment—administrators, concerned faculty, dormitory staff, and university public safety officers—should be aware of the importance of maintaining confidentiality, but also the importance of breaking confidentiality in an emergency. In addition to confidentiality of patient records, another unique confidentiality issue can occur with parents, families, or significant others contacting the mental health service out of their concern for student-patients. Legal guidelines must be negotiated with university counsel, administration, and student government leaders, and made available to all students on a proactive basis, as well as when students become patients.

Lines of responsibility. College mental health services are usually located within a student health service, with the psychiatrist reporting administratively to the latter's director or to the vice-president for student affairs. Consideration should be given to having the health service report directly to the medical school dean, if possible.

When psychiatrists are administrators of college mental health services, they can organize intake procedures, therapy responsibilities, emergency coverage, and supervision along psychiatric models. When they function as consultants or staff psychiatrists, with others in administrative roles, they must negotiate clear lines of reporting and responsibility.

Legal issues. Psychiatrists must ensure that all their college and university mental health colleagues understand that legal responsibility, with the hazard of malpractice suits, rests with the psychiatrist who is most trained in general medicine and all areas of mental health and illness.

Unique and Rewarding Opportunities in Psychiatry in a University Setting

Treating a challenging, diverse population. Treating college and university students today offers energetic, well-trained psychiatrists numerous challenges for many reasons. First among these is the increasing age span of students, from their late teenage years to their

60s and even beyond, especially in urban settings. A second change among the student population is the increasing complexity of their personal and family histories, including incredible experiences of trauma and complicated psychiatric illnesses. Students reach a point where they feel compelled to seek consultation and treatment because they can no longer deny and contain their symptoms when these begin to interfere with their academic and extracurricular functioning.

Unquestionably, for psychiatrists who choose to practice in the college setting, opportunities abound to interact with a challenging, intelligent group of people of increasingly diverse ages, backgrounds, and personal problems. In this setting, one is easily and frequently inspired by the personal strengths, energy, and potential for healing and growth among our future citizens, professionals, and community and national leaders. By the same token, college psychiatrists trained to deal with patients' seemingly insurmountable personal trauma and severe chronic mental illnesses are often aghast but simultaneously challenged to help students face and work through previous destructive experiences while the students simultaneously attempt to meet rigorous academic requirements successfully.

Professional growth opportunities. Between the 1970s and mid-1980s, college psychiatry flourished, with many full-time psychiatrists involved in student treatment. The mental health section of the American College Health Association, a national organization of school and individual members of all health and mental health disciplines, founded in 1920, has held excellent annual programs. Issues are raised and research data and model treatment programs are presented to interested attendees. Attendees gain as much from informal networking across mental health and health specialties and across geographic and school borders as they do from the formal programs. The multidisciplinary *Journal of American College Health* includes research and clinical papers concerning student mental health issues and successful programs.

Flexible work schedule. Work hours can be very flexible, particularly for those who work part-time. The psychiatrist's presence at weekly staff conferences is usually firmly arranged, but consultation hours with student-patients and supervision of staff can often be negotiated to mesh with other responsibilities.

For physicians with young children who want to be more available to family at certain hours, college psychiatry can be a satisfying and manageable professional opportunity.

Personal rewards. The gratitude students feel for the help they receive is extremely rewarding, whether expressed indirectly in their academic and relationship successes or directly through notes, cards, and office visits soon after therapy ends or years later. Hearing or reading about one's former student-patients' successes in careers and in personal life experiences, or meeting them in airports and stopping to catch up, are immeasurably satisfying and unexpected rewards.

Financial and Practical Considerations

At most mental health facilities, students are charged for services. All students should have health insurance that includes mental health coverage to ensure availability of care to all. Psychiatrists should press universities to mandate health insurance to cover needed inpatient care as well as the more commonly necessary outpatient medical evaluation, including the physical examination and laboratory workups necessary before psychiatric or other medication is prescribed. To assume that young adults are healthy and do not require such evaluation is dangerous, as even athlete-patients can have cardiac abnormalities on electrocardiograms and require further workup. When hospitalization becomes a necessity, procedures must also be in place to arrange for transportation to local, state, or regional facilities.

College psychiatrists receive salaries on a yearly or contractual basis. If they are psychiatry department faculty members, they must meet promotion and tenure or clinical track requirements. When a practitioner is the only psychiatrist at a college, he or she must arrange night and weekend emergency coverage. (For coverage, students are also given the university hospital's 24-hour emergency psychiatry telephone number.)

Conclusion: The Future of College and University Mental Health

In 1993, an increasing number of psychiatrists reverted to part-time consulting roles with college and university health services and, less frequently, with counseling centers, as increasing fiscal constraints and changing university policies delegated full-time positions to other mental health professionals. Nevertheless, psychiatrists will always be needed on college campuses as professional team leaders, consultants, and, if time and finances permit, therapists for individuals, couples, and groups.

References

Blain D: Women in psychiatry, in National Commission on Mental Health Manpower Careers in Psychiatry. Edited by Burch C, Van Atta W, Blain D. New York, Macmillan, 1968, pp 111–127

Dickstein LJ: Social change and dependency in university men: the white knight complex unresolved. J College Student Psychotherapy 1:31–41, 1986

Farnsworth D: Psychiatry, Education, and the Young Adult. Springfield, IL, Charles C Thomas, 1966

Glasscote R, Fishman M: Mental Health on Campus: A Field Study. Washington, DC, American Psychiatric Press, 1973

Talley JE, Rockwell WJ: Counseling and Psychotherapy Services for University Students. Springfield, IL, Charles C Thomas, 1985

Whittington HG: Psychiatry on the College Campus. New York, International Universities Press, 1963

Section II:
Setting-Related Careers

Organized Care Practice

CHAPTER ELEVEN

Health Maintenance Organization Psychiatry

Judith L. Feldman, M.D.

A Brief History of HMOs

The first health maintenance organizations (HMOs) were physician-dominated, staff-model organizations. Many of them did not offer mental health care or else offered it only as an optional rider (Bittker 1985). As managed care proved profitable, a plethora of other models developed. These include group models, where a practice group contracts with a managed care organization, and independent practice associations (IPAs), where individual physicians form—and pay to join—an association and have a part of their usual fee withheld to be returned to them based on the performance of the organization. Other IPAs, or group model HMOs, pay physicians or practice groups a *capitation fee* (price per head fee) to care for each patient in a panel, out of which the physician or group have to purchase laboratory tests and specialty care. Specialists, including mental health clinicians, are generally paid on a fee-for-service basis out of this capitation allowance. Some organizations developed *carve-out* arrangements, in which all mental health care is sent to a particular group of practitioners, which might or might not include a psychiatrist. Clinicians also formed preferred provider organizations (PPOs). Patients can go to a PPO practitioner or to anyone in the community for covered care, but receive better coverage or lower copayments with the PPO. In exchange for this advantage, PPO providers agree to low fees or more cost-effective practices.

In parallel with the development of these care systems came the development of *utilization review* and *utilization management companies* (i.e., companies that contract with employers, insurance companies, or HMOs to "manage" aspects of care) (Rodriguez 1992). These arrangements have become very popular in the mental health field, as neither employers nor HMO managers had clear ideas about how to manage mental health costs, which were increasing steadily in all treatment settings.

A Career With a Health Maintenance Organization

It is clear from the above that there is a wide variety of career possibilities within the field of managed care. Psychiatrists may contract with IPAs, develop and work in PPOs, perform utilization reviews and manage utilization review companies, or work as HMO employees. I will focus primarily on the staff-model HMO, as that is the type of place where I have had the most direct clinical and administrative experience.

Staff-model HMOs originated in the 1940s from attempts of organized labor to obtain coverage for workers (Bennett 1988). They use limited resources to serve a defined population, and employ salaried mental health staff of many disciplines, organized into departments usually within a multispecialty medical institution. They have become part of a large, private managed care movement and serve mainly an employer-based membership. HMOs serve the severely ill only as part of a broad spectrum of patients, and often exclude chronic illness from coverage. They are almost totally prepaid, collecting only a small revenue from copayments. The HMO is the insurer as well as the system that delivers the care.

In the rest of this chapter, I outline some of the major opportunities and problems posed by staff-model HMOs as settings for psychiatric practice and discuss these as they influence work and practice conditions for clinicians.

I began working for a staff-model HMO in Boston, Massachusetts, in 1974, when it had 40,000 members and two sites. (It currently has more than 560,000 members and 65 sites!) Within this HMO, I have been a staff psychiatrist in an outpatient department and a day hospital, a chief of a mental health department, and an associate chief of hospital-based services; I have done research, teaching, and supervision, and have directed continuing education courses.

A large managed care organization offers a wide variety of opportunities. Some of the advantages of academia (e.g., collegial support; opportunities for continuing education, teaching, researching, and writing; sometimes tenure) are available without the pressure to publish. There is also a wide range of clinical possibilities. Most HMOs enroll a wide range of members in terms of their age, degree of illness, type of problem, socioeconomic status, and background. There is a large enough population base to run group programs and to develop specialty services. The HMO for which I work currently has a behavioral medicine program, a day hospital, a chronic care program, an eating disorders program, an incest survivors program, a substance abuse program, and a consultation service. There are opportunities to work collegially with other mental health professionals and with physicians in all specialties (Schneider-Braus 1987).

The Fundamental Conflict

A fundamental conflict underlies all work in an HMO that makes the work challenging, interesting, and constantly bordering on unethical. Any physician working as the employee of an HMO has allegiances to a patient, to a group of patients, to the patient's employer (who may be paying for the health coverage), and to the HMO, which not only provides the health care but also insures it (Hartig and Eichelman 1986). The implications of this conflict reach every corner and invade every moment of practice in an HMO. Implications of this conflict include the following (Feldman 1992):

1. Any patient who has prepaid his or her health coverage feels "entitled" to care. This feeling is particularly keen in the mental health field, where care may be experienced as desirable or pleasurable, as well as necessary, and is further amplified in some patients with character disorders.
2. A salaried practitioner does not receive additional money for seeing additional patients. The HMO strives to hire the minimum effective number of practitioners and to keep them busy. Therefore, a

clinician must think not only of the patient currently in the office, but also of the patients who are "out there" waiting to come in, and of his or her fixed schedule. The clinician is motivated to limit care, and the patient to extend it—to the limits of coverage. This puts the patient and the clinician potentially in conflict.
3. Organizational goals usually center around keeping costs down, retaining current members, and marketing to new ones. These goals may sometimes conflict with the clinical goals of providing quality care and advocating for the patient. In particular, setting appropriate limits on an acting-out or substance-abusing patient may result in the patient's complaining to an administrator, and, in some cases, the undermining of a therapeutic intervention.
4. As psychiatrists become involved in administrative or clinical decisions in organizations that provide financial incentives based on productivity or cost, they are at risk for making cost-based decisions as agents of their employer rather than of their patients (Sederer and St. Clair 1989).

Consequences for Clinical Practice

HMOs vary tremendously in their ability to balance the aforementioned factors and simultaneously support clinicians in an optimal managed care practice. Ideally, an organization should be managed by individuals with some understanding of mental health care, the need for appropriate resources, and the support of clinicians. In turn, clinicians who work in an HMO ideally should be concerned with a public health model of care in which care is given from a pool of limited resources to a group of patients. The care should be of high quality and satisfying to the individual patient, but should use the most parsimonious method effective in each clinical situation (Van Buskirk et al. 1985).

Sabin (1991) wrote about six crucial skills that can help clinicians meet the demands of HMO practice:

- Population-oriented practice management
- Population-oriented program development

- Ability to apply an adult developmental model
- Command of a broad repertoire of methodology
- Ethical analysis
- Advocacy

To these I would add:

- Ability to understand and work within complex systems of care
- Ability to develop and use treatment guidelines and algorithms
- Differential therapeutics and treatment planning
- Patience
- A sense of humor

Many organizations fall short of this ideal. However, the popular myths about HMOs (e.g., "HMOs don't provide psychiatric care." "HMOs offer only group therapy and crisis intervention." "HMOs treat only healthy patients." "HMOs don't employ psychiatrists.") are generally untrue.

The mental health program and benefits offered by an HMO depend in large part on the state-mandated mental health benefits and whether they apply to HMOs in that state (American Psychiatric Association 1986). For example, in Massachusetts there is a mandated benefit of $500 of outpatient care and 60 days of psychiatric inpatient care without exclusions. This means that an HMO must offer care to all patients regardless of diagnosis or chronicity. Because the HMO must cover up to 60 days of (costly) inpatient care, it often offers more than the usual maximum of 20 outpatient sessions to chronic patients to try to avert hospitalization. An HMO in a state without mandated benefits could choose to offer no psychiatric benefits, or could offer benefits that exclude patients with certain conditions or diagnoses.

Being an Employee

In addition to the conflicts detailed above, there are other considerations involved in adopting employee status. Psychiatrist-employees have limited control over their practices. In most HMOs, psychiatrists cannot say no to treating a patient, must do what is needed in the department, and have little control over hiring administrative and other support staff or over choosing the type of medical record used or paperwork required. There may be productivity standards, and there surely will be periodic performance reviews.

However, salary is guaranteed, benefits generally are quite good and include vacation and maternity leave, and the institution assumes some legal liability. Night call is shared; there is ready collegiality and time and money for continued education.

Who Should Work in an HMO?

It is probably clear at this point that the care delivered in an HMO tends to brief, focused, goal oriented, active, and eclectic. Although psychiatrists may have long relationships with some patients, these relationships often rely on the structure of the HMO and the primary physician as providing a "holding environment" and consist of intermittent visits or brief episodes of care (Cummings 1991). Skills in evaluation and differential treatment planning are essential, but are usually not well taught in training programs. Ideally, a psychiatrist should be able to "shift gears" rapidly, doing a medication evaluation with one patient, followed by hypnosis with another, brief dynamic treatment with a third, then a group session, a consultation with an internist, and so forth. The pace of practice is rapid and there is often little time for reflection. Psychiatrists often manage a large number of chronically ill patients and should enjoy working with a team of other mental health colleagues.

In evaluating an HMO as a potential work setting, psychiatrists must first establish that basic standards of practice are possible. For example, they should ask the following questions: Are psychiatrists able to do face-to-face evaluations of every patient for whom they prescribe medication? Do psychiatrists have adequate time to document encounters with patients or to supervise other mental health clinicians? Toward these ends, in 1989 the American Psychiatric Association approved a set of guidelines entitled "Guidelines for Psychiatric Practice in Staff Model HMOs." A copy is available through the American

Psychiatric Association and may be helpful to psychiatrists evaluating HMOs as potential workplaces.

Conclusion

A colleague in my state psychiatric society once asked me to give a talk on my "alternative lifestyle." She was not referring to beads, sandals, or folk music, but to my career in an HMO. My colleagues in fee-for-service practice sometimes view me with suspicion, as someone who has sold out, who threatens their financial security, or who has compromised her standards of care. There are certainly some real differences in political outlook between salaried and fee-for-service practitioners. (For example, an increase in state-mandated mental health benefits would be a delight to a private practitioner. To an HMO psychiatrist, it might just mean an increase in patient entitlement without an increase in organizational resources to provide the care.) However, as utilization review organizations and employer self-insurance plans proliferate, and as public psychiatry becomes more "managed," there are fewer real differences between us. We are all trying to manage, with a limited pot of money, to provide the best possible care. For the right person, an HMO is an exciting and challenging setting in which to provide this patient care.

References

American Psychiatric Association: Section IV (Coverage for Psychiatric Illnesses in HMOs), in The Coverage Catalog. Washington, DC, American Psychiatric Press, 1986, pp 375–403

American Psychiatric Association, Task Force on Professional Practice Issues in Managed Care Systems: Guidelines for Psychiatric Practice in Staff Model HMOs. Washington, DC, APA, June 1989

Bennett MJ: The greening of the HMO: implications for prepaid psychiatry. Am J Psychiatry 145:1544–1549, 1988

Bittker TE: The industrialization of American psychiatry. Am J Psychiatry 142:149–154, 1985

Cummings N: Brief intermittent therapy throughout the life cycle, in Psychotherapy in Managed Health Care. Edited by Austad C, Berman W. Washington, DC, American Psychological Association, 1991, pp 35–46

Feldman JL: The managed care setting and the patient-therapist relationship, in Managed Mental Health Care: Administrative and Clinical Issues. Edited by Feldman JL, Fitzpatrick R. Washington, DC, American Psychiatric Press, 1992, pp 219–230

Hartig A, Eichelman B: The ethics of mental health practice. Psychiatric Annals 16:547–552, 1986

Rodriguez AR: Management of quality, utilization, and risk, in Managed Mental Health Care: Administrative and Clinical Issues. Edited by Feldman JL, Fitzpatrick R. Washington, DC, American Psychiatric Press, 1992, pp 83–89

Sabin JE: Clinical skills for the 1990s: six lessons from HMO practice. Hosp Community Psychiatry 42:605–608, 1991

Schneider-Braus K: A practical guide to HMO psychiatry. Hosp Community Psychiatry 38:876–879, 1987

Sederer LI, St. Clair L: Managed health care and the Massachusetts experience. Am J Psychiatry 146:1142–1148, 1989

Van Buskirk D, Feldman JL, Steinberg S, et al: Teaching psychiatry in the health maintenance organization. Am J Psychiatry 142:1181–1183, 1985

CHAPTER TWELVE

Community Psychiatry

Gordon H. Clark, Jr., M.D.

A Brief History of Community Mental Health Centers

The idealistic aim of the community mental health center (CMHC) movement, initiated in the Kennedy administration in the early 1960s, was to provide coordinated psychiatric services to large numbers of people in their own communities. Although psychiatrists were initially mandated by regulations to be in charge of CMHCs, subsequent regulations eliminated this requirement. Other mental health professionals assumed more and more patient care and administrative responsibilities. That CMHCs developed in an era of social pressures toward equality, as evidenced by the civil rights and women's movements, undoubtedly contributed to the role blurring that has been variously described as *functional egalitarianism* (Eaton and Goldstein 1977), *pseudo-egalitarianism* (Langsley and Barter 1983), *false egalitarianism* (Borus 1978), *expedient deprofessionalization* (Ruiz and Tourlentes 1983), and an *orgy of role transvestism* (Freedman 1978). Also plagued by inadequate training opportunities, salaries, and status, many competent psychiatrists felt compelled to withdraw from CMHCs because they were not granted authority commensurate with their medicolegal responsibility. Concomitantly, concerns developed regarding both deterioration in the quality of care provided by these centers (Arce and Vergare 1985; Freedman 1978; Perr 1986) and apparent abandonment of their original mission; as stated in a report by the Group for the Advancement of Psychiatry (1983), "for the most part CMHCs are not taking adequate care of the seriously and chronically mentally ill patients" (p. 3).

In response to these concerns, the American Association of Community Mental Health Psychiatrists (AACMHP) was founded in 1984 (it became the American Association of Community Psychiatrists [AACP] in 1987) with the goals of providing mutual support for community psychiatrists, clearly defining the community psychiatrist's role (with responsibility linked to authority), enhancing the quality and quantity of training and research in community psychiatry, increasing the recruitment and retention of competent community psychiatrists, and, ultimately, upgrading both the quality of care within CMHCs and the image of community psychiatry. Through the efforts of the AACP's dedicated members, there has been a resurgence of interest in community psychiatry. Inroads have begun toward changes that allow community psychiatrists to fulfill their ideals by practicing in these challenging settings without having to compromise their personal or professional values. DuMas, a psychologist, predicted in 1974 that CMHCs would, after passing through nonmedical and then antimedical models, return to a medical model of patient care:

> In the long run this transition should be good for medical and nonmedical health practitioners as well as the general public, and out of these uncomfortable adjustments will come a better program of community health care. (p. 878)

A Career in Community Psychiatry

Community psychiatry may well offer the prospective practitioner the greatest variety of experiences available within the field of psychiatry. There is variety in terms of age of patients cared for, spectrum and severity of illnesses seen, and socioeconomic groups served. There is variety in terms of treatment sites: outpatient clinics, emergency rooms, inpatient psychiatric units and medical-surgical units, partial hospital programs, homes of patients and family members, group homes, nursing homes, shelters, police stations, and jails. Indeed, the CMHC, now somewhat of an anachronism, is only one of a number of settings in which one may practice community psychiatry. There is variety in terms of collaborators, including other clinicians (both in and out of the agency), members of the state's department of mental health, members of the judiciary, and members of the local chapters of advocacy groups, such as the National Alliance for the Mentally Ill. There is variety in the roles to be fulfilled in the community setting:

clinician, supervisor, teacher, and administrator. Finally, in comprehensively attending to patients' biopsychosocial needs, there is variety in terms of applied treatment modalities: somatic therapies; individual, couple, family, and group therapies; behavioral strategies; and psychosocial rehabilitative applications.

There is also wide variation, as suggested earlier, in how community programs are managed, in the quality of clinical care they deliver, and in how they are experienced by psychiatrists. Some are doing an excellent job and have little difficulty recruiting and retaining competent psychiatrists.

In a national survey of community psychiatrists (Clark and Vaccaro 1987), respondents noted several factors that seemed to contribute to job satisfaction:

- Having a variety of tasks to perform
- Being valued for possessing uniquely comprehensive expertise and performing a clinical oversight role
- Serving as a center's executive director
- Working in a CMHC that is integrally tied to a hospital or academic institution

Role of Psychiatrists in CMHCs: The Central Problem

In 1971, 55% of CMHCs had psychiatrists as executive directors (Dewey and Astrachan 1985). By 1985, this figure had dropped dramatically to 8% (Knox 1985); in 1995 there are doubtless even fewer. Psychiatrists do not possess unique administrative skills any more than they possess unique psychotherapeutic skills. Although it may not be necessary to have a psychiatrist as the executive director, it is essential, in any given community psychiatric program, to have a medical director whose role is clearly defined and supported. When this does not happen, the psychiatrist is generally expected to assume medicolegal responsibility without being granted commensurate clinical authority. Such untenable situations ultimately lead to a demise in the quality of both the center's psychiatric staff and its clinical care.

In community settings where the role of psychiatry is not adequately defined or supported, psychiatrists may experience a variety of difficulties. In the aforementioned national survey of community psychiatrists (Clark and Vaccaro 1987), respondents identified 10 factors that contributed to job dissatisfaction and burnout (most of these seemed to reflect directly both an inadequate definition of and support for the role of the psychiatrist):

- Having a lack of administrative support and validation
- Receiving no recognition for board certification
- Having responsibility for the work of other staff without authority or time to supervise them adequately
- Being restricted to a single task (e.g., only evaluating patients for medication)
- Feeling pressure to sign documents related to patients whom they have no part in treating
- Feeling pressure to see more patients in less time
- Having excessive amounts of paperwork
- Feeling a lack of respect from psychiatrists and physicians outside the CMHC
- Receiving low pay
- Feeling in conflict with the CMHC's mission (i.e., when there is overemphasis on social as opposed to medical services)

Personal Considerations

As in other organized care settings, psychiatrists working in community psychiatric programs do not have control over their time, choice of patients, or supports for the practices. They may feel the pinch of budget shortfalls or the consequences of poor or inefficient management. However, as is also true in other organized settings, psychiatrists in community settings have the advantages of a salary (on-call time is generally reimbursed extra), paid vacation and holidays, health and disability coverage (life and dental coverage may also be included), and generally some form of retirement plan. Paid leave for continuing medical education (ideally with additional funding for travel, meals, lodging, and educational costs) and malpractice insurance coverage are generally provided. However, because these last two have been problem areas for psychiatrists in some community programs, the prospective community psychiatrist should ensure that these are provided at adequate levels.

Current Initiatives in Community Psychiatry

Among the basic principles of community psychiatry are accessibility, comprehensiveness of services, treatment in the least restrictive alternative, and continuity of care.

- *Accessibility* means being proximally and immediately available for patients in crisis.
- *Comprehensiveness* means diagnosing and treating patients biopsychosocially, and tailoring the array of services available within community systems to individual needs and choices (Stein et al. 1990).
- *Treatment in the least restrictive alternative* means affording the patient as much freedom and responsibility for his or her own care as possible; thus, treatment in the least restrictive alternative really becomes treatment in the most therapeutic alternative.
- *Continuity of care* means providing as much consistency of caregivers for each patient as possible.

Toward these ideals, there have been the following recent developments in community psychiatric programs: mobile crisis teams that provide immediate access to patients experiencing psychiatric emergencies, assertive community treatment teams that provide continuity of care through mobile outreach, and innovative psychosocial rehabilitative models that strive to reduce disability and restore maximal functioning. Community psychiatrists are in the forefront of advocacy efforts on behalf of psychiatric patients who have acquired immunodeficiency syndrome (Goldfinger 1990) or are homeless (Lamb et al. 1992). Community psychiatrists are also ardent advocates for universal access to health care, with parity for psychiatric conditions.

Although funding can certainly be a problem in some states and for some community programs, new initiatives continue to emerge, such as those by the Robert Wood Johnson Foundation, aiming toward greater integration of services (Shore and Cohen 1990), and by the Pew Memorial Trust, aiming toward greater state and university collaboration (Talbott 1991).

CMHCs and other community psychiatric programs have increasingly been called upon to function as part of a system. According to Talbott (1983), an ideal system requires

1) a clear separation between planning and implementation,
2) point responsibility for a specific population, with one person in charge and all services administratively responsible to one person,
3) clinical integration at the lowest level of government,
4) elimination of both competition between elements in the system for elite patients and neglect of undesirable patients,
5) elimination of duplications and gaps in services,
6) elimination of communication difficulties,
7) tracking mechanisms for patients, and
8) a single funding mechanism.
(p. 16)

Community psychiatrists are actively engaged in system design and implementation at all levels: within their own programs, ensuring timely, appropriate, and coordinated treatment; within the communities, integrating patient-client services with those provided by other agencies; within their regions, interfacing with state hospitals regarding patient admissions and discharges; within their states, collaborating with state offices of mental health to ensure adequate funding and appropriate programming and staffing; and at a national level, networking with the following entities:

- Funding bodies—such as the National Institute of Mental Health
- Political bodies—such as the National Association of State Mental Health Program Directors and the National Council of Community Mental Health Centers
- Consumer organizations—such as the National Mental Health

Consumers Association and the National Association of Psychiatric Survivors
- Advocacy organizations—such as the National Alliance for the Mentally Ill and the National Mental Health Association
- Accrediting bodies—such as the Joint Commission on Accreditation of Healthcare Organizations and the Commission on Accreditation of Rehabilitation Facilities
- Professional organizations—such as the AACP and the American Psychiatric Association (APA)

Who Should Work in a CMHC or Other Community Psychiatric Program?

Psychiatrists considering a career in a community setting should certainly have a good measure of social idealism and a desire to serve their community, along with interest and skill in treating patients with serious mental disorders in a variety of settings. They should have had the benefit of a quality training experience with competent and committed community psychiatric role models. Prospective community psychiatrists should enjoy working with other professionals on a multidisciplinary team and be as clear as possible about their own standards of medical practice. The "Guidelines for Psychiatric Practice in Community Mental Health Centers" (American Psychiatric Association 1991), approved by both the AACP and the APA, is a good yardstick by which to judge whether a given community psychiatric program will be supportive of one's standards and allow one to practice comfortably in that particular setting.

Clearly, there has been a tremendous resurgence of interest among psychiatrists in community psychiatry. The work is exciting, challenging, and gratifying. Community psychiatric programs are the front lines where, thanks to multidisciplinary teams, one's psychiatric expertise can have a broad ripple effect, with a positive impact on the lives of a great many individuals and families who struggle with the often devastating consequences of serious mental illness. More and more residents just out of training, as well as other psychiatrists, seem to be attracted to community programs. There are more good models available now of how community programs may optimally be structured and operated. There are more university training programs in community psychiatry for residents and fellows. There is now an organization, the AACP, to provide collegial support and to serve as a collective voice, advocating for quality patient care, for appropriate utilization of the community psychiatrist's comprehensive expertise, and for effective training and research initiatives.

Although the "bugs" are not fully out of the community psychiatry system, certainly tremendous headway has been and is being made. This is an exciting time to be part of a renewed, collective effort toward realizing the original dream envisioned by President Kennedy in the Community Mental Health Act of 1963.

Conclusion

Since the inception of the community mental health movement in the early 1960s, community psychiatrists have faced many challenges. This is largely because they have been isolated from each other and therefore more vulnerable to abuse in problematic community settings. However, the wrongs have not all been on one side. Some psychiatrists have used CMHCs merely as stepping-stones into private practice. The community psychiatrists who have come together to create the AACP are dedicated to ensuring that quality medicine can be practiced in community mental health settings and that psychiatrists can have lasting careers in these settings. Toward these ends, the AACP is engaged in actively supporting its members, providing continuing education programs, developing model training curricula, promoting research, and collaborating with a host of other organizations. Not since CMHCs came into being has community psychiatry held the promise it holds today.

References

American Psychiatric Association: Guidelines for psychiatric practice in community mental health centers. Am J Psychiatry 148:965–966, 1991

Arce AA, Vergare MJ: Psychiatrists and interprofessional role conflicts in community mental health centers, in Community Mental Health Centers and Psychiatrists. Edited by a Joint Steering Committee of the American Psychiatric Association and the National Council of Community Mental Health Centers. Washington, DC, American Psychiatric Association, 1985, pp 51–68

Borus JF: Critical to the survival of community mental health. Am J Psychiatry 135:1029–1035, 1978

Clark GH, Vaccaro JV: Burnout among CMHC psychiatrists and the struggle to survive. Hosp Community Psychiatry 38:843–847, 1987

Community Mental Health Act of 1963, Public Law 88-164

Dewey L, Astrachan BM: Organizational issues in recruitment and retention of psychiatrists by CMHCs, in Community Mental Health Centers and Psychiatrists. Edited by a Joint Steering Committee of the American Psychiatric Association and the National Council of Community Mental Health Centers. Washington, DC, American Psychiatric Association, 1985, pp 22–31

DuMas FM: Medical, nonmedical or antimedical modes for mental health centers? Am J Psychiatry 131:875–878, 1974

Eaton JS, Goldstein LS: Psychiatry in crisis. Am J Psychiatry 134:642–645, 1977

Freedman DX: Community mental health: slogan and a history of the mission, in Controversy in Psychiatry. Edited by Brady JP, Brodie HKH. Philadelphia, PA, WB Saunders, 1978, pp 1060–1070

Goldfinger SM (ed): Psychiatric Aspects of AIDS and HIV Infection. New Directions for Mental Health Services, No. 48. San Francisco, CA, Jossey-Bass, 1990

Group for the Advancement of Psychiatry, Committee on Psychiatry and Community: Community Psychiatry: A Reappraisal. New York, Mental Health Materials Center, 1983

Knox MD: National registry reveals profile of service provider. National Council News 9:1, 1985

Lamb HR, Bachrach LL, Kass FI (eds): Treating the Homeless Mentally Ill. Washington, DC, American Psychiatric Press, 1992

Langsley DG, Barter JT: Psychiatric roles in the community mental health center. Hosp Community Psychiatry 34:729–733, 1983

Perr IN: New multitier system in psychiatry. Psychiatric Times 3:2:1, 12, 14, 19, February 1986

Ruiz P, Tourlentes TT: Community mental health centers, in Psychiatric Administration. Edited by Talbott JA, Kaplan SR. New York, Grune & Stratton, 1983, pp 103–119

Shore MS, Cohen MD: The Robert Wood Johnson Program on Chronic Mental Illness: an overview. Hosp Community Psychiatry 41:1212–1216, 1990

Stein LI, Diamond RJ, Factor RM: A systems approach to the care of persons with schizophrenia, in Handbook of Schizophrenia, Vol 5 (Psychosocial Therapies). Edited by Herz MI, Keith SJ, Docherty JP. Amsterdam, The Netherlands, Elsevier Science Publishers, 1990, pp 213–246

Talbott JA: Trends in the delivery of psychiatric services, in Psychiatric Administration. Edited by Talbott JA, Kaplan SR. New York, Grune & Stratton, 1983, pp 3–19

Talbott JA (ed): State University Collaboration Project: collected articles. Hosp Community Psychiatry 42:39–73, 1991

CHAPTER THIRTEEN

Military Psychiatry

Maria E. Esposito, M.D.
Robert J. Ursano, M.D.[1]

Introduction

> Whether or not we wish it, war continues to be part of the human experience; and the military represents a significant force in the scheme of things. Acknowledging that reality, [it] behooves us to increase the contributions psychiatry can make in this area. (Menninger 1987, p. 3)

The military community has over 10 million members, including active duty and retired service personnel and their families. The community spans the world, from the United States to Europe and the Far East, and includes members living afloat in European and Asian waters (Ursano 1987; Ursano and Holloway 1985; Ursano et al. 1989).[2] The Medical Corps was established as part of the United States military on July 27, 1775, with the appointment of the first Director General and Chief Physician (Crocker 1981).

In this chapter, we focus on career opportunities for the psychiatrist who is also a uniformed military medical corps officer, and describe the unique challenges inherent to living and practicing in the military community. We hope to assist interested medical students, interns, and civilian psychiatrists eligible for appointment to the Armed Forces

---

[1] This work was done as part of our employment by the federal government and is, therefore, in the public domain. The opinions expressed are those of the authors and do not necessarily reflect the views of the Department of Defense or the Uniformed Services University of the Health Sciences School of Medicine.

[2] These three references by Ursano and colleagues provide the source for many facts and views in this chapter and will not be specifically cited in each instance. The reader is alerted to them for further reading on the subject of the chapter.

in making an informed and intelligent career choice.

Military psychiatrists are male and female uniformed military officers whose patients come from the entire military community. They work in their chosen branch of the service, providing primary, secondary, and tertiary preventive services via consultation, direct clinical care, education, and research.

What does a military psychiatrist do? Your day could begin with lending your expertise in a telemedicine space bridge, consulting via satellite with pediatric psychiatrists in Armenia who are dealing with earthquake victims. Here you might be asked to interview and discuss the case of a 15-year-old female who sustained multiple injuries in the 1988 earthquake, as well as give specific information about psychopharmacology and posttraumatic stress disorder (PTSD). This may be followed by a request from the local school district to evaluate a family in which the active duty father, an Army sergeant, has died from complications of acquired immunodeficiency syndrome (AIDS); his wife is depressed and is having difficulty coping with her loss, and their four children are having behavioral problems. Soon after completing the family evaluation, you might be asked to see an active duty sailor who became anxious after receiving orders to report for submarine duty.

If you are assigned to a general medical hospital that is also a teaching facility, you will be responsible for supervising medical students and psychiatry residents. While supervising the therapy of a severely borderline patient, you may be interrupted by another resident who asks to consult with you on three outpatient emergencies: the first, an Air Force officer with marital problems who became severely depressed as his first son prepared to leave for college; the second, a referral from a local unit of a new recruit who is hearing the voice of his dead grandmother; and finally, a soldier's wife referred from the emergency room with severe abdominal pain whose symptoms developed 24 hours after her husband left for an unaccompanied assignment in Somalia. When assigned to an operational unit, you may, during a typical day, respond to a call from the commander seeking guidance on handling a young enlisted soldier who is crying, "I will kill myself if I can't get out of the military and go home!"

Military psychiatry can be viewed as a subspecialty with identifiable knowledge and skills. The military psychiatrist must be familiar with the specific stressors and psychosocial context of the community in which he or she practices. Community psychiatry and consultation-liaison psychiatry are the basis of the military psychiatrist's activities. Community psychiatry offers a wide variety of responsibilities and roles to a psychiatrist. It focuses on direct clinical care delivery as well as indirect care, including administrative functions, consultative responsibilities, research, and educational tasks. Military psychiatrists provide both direct and indirect services. As direct caregivers, they treat patients with all types and severity of illnesses, in ambulatory and hospital care, following a biopsychosocial approach. In addition, the military psychiatrist is prepared to organize and deliver a wide range of indirect services in a variety of military settings, working with professionals and nonprofessionals including administrators, consultants, educators, and researchers.

The Role of the Psychiatrist in the Military Community

Understanding the military community is very important to accurately portraying the responsibility of a typical psychiatric medical officer. Such an officer could be stationed in the United States or overseas, live on military installations, and work with uniformed and non-uniformed personnel. The military is a total community environment with hospitals, housing, schools, social clubs, and recreational facilities. Military psychiatrists' work settings are defined by their branch of service and duty assignment. They must know how service members organize their lives; what stressors occur in operational settings, during training, in garrison (peacetime), or on battlefields (wartime); and what places service members and their families at risk for emotional and physical disease. A service member's illness can jeopardize not only his or her individual health and performance, but potentially that of his or her co-workers in performing their mission. The services provided by psychiatrists include not only individual assessments and treatment, but also prevention and consultation at all levels of the organizational structure.

As part of the military community, military psychiatrists also treat families and retirees, including over 2 million children and adolescent dependents, approximately 90% of whom are under age 13. One or both parents may be on active duty and some may be single parents; single parents have to function as both service members and parents (Belenky 1987). The psychiatrist must be attuned to the nuances of this community. Boredom, substance abuse, anxiety disorders, and family and military stressors can exacerbate preexisting personality disorders or precipitate major psychiatric disorders.

As with many large organizations, military service members are required to travel and be assigned overseas on temporary assignments, as well as for 3- or 4-year tours. Some are isolated tours of 1 year's duration, requiring separation from family and friends. Geographic moves, whether for the individual service member or for the entire family, offer unique opportunities as well as potential for emotional and family disturbances.

After a 20- or 30-year career, while only in midlife, a service member faces retirement, requiring him or her to make new career decisions while mourning the loss of the military career. This period can be a stressful one, necessitating support programs to help with the transition.

Direct Clinical Care Delivery

In their day-to-day practice, military psychiatrists work with active duty service members, their families, and retirees. Members of this community face the unique stressors of their community as well as crises similar to those in civilian communities, such as separations, divorce, single parenthood, dual-working parents, and retirement. Soldiers, sailors, airmen and airwomen, and their families are constantly anticipating the possibility of separations for short and long tours of duty, isolated tours, and frequent geographic moves while faced with the constant potential for war and death. Isolated tours for submarine duty last 3 to 12 months with only rare communication from family, possibly an occasional "familygram." These missions include the stress of isolation, confinement, sleep deprivation, rigid schedules, and boredom. Entire families experience frequent moves away from their families of origin to areas of different cultures and languages. In one recently treated family, the adolescent, a senior in high school, complained of having been in eight different schools before he reached 10th grade.

Military psychiatrists, as direct caregivers, evaluate and treat inpatients and outpatients, providing a full range of services: crisis intervention; behavioral, group, marital, and family therapy; and insight-oriented psychotherapy. In wartime, care is focused on treatment of combat psychiatric casualties, using the principles of brevity, immediacy, centrality, expectancy, proximity, and simplicity. These principles of care facilitate individuals' return to their units (Belenky 1987). In past wars, 85% of casualties have been returned to duty when these principles of crisis intervention and prevention were used. These techniques inhibit regressive behaviors, leading to fewer relapses, and ultimately lessen the chronicity of psychiatric symptoms.

Military Psychiatrists as Consultants

As consultants in the military, community military psychiatrists fill various capacities in peacetime and in war. Unit commanders play a large role in contributing to service members' sense of well-being and unit cohesion. For this reason, military psychiatrists form a close relationship with the hierarchical command structure to monitor morale. Military psychiatrists provide support and education to facilitate combat readiness while decreasing personal conflicts. Absent without leave (AWOL) rates, drug abuse, and other forms of disturbing behavior are related to the degree of stress on a military unit (Belenky 1987). Consultation frequently helps identify whether a particular problem is unique to an individual service member or reflects an ongoing group stress.

At times, military psychiatrists are asked to evaluate individuals for "fitness for duty." Major psychiatric disorders are causes for separation or medical retirement, and other conditions may limit access to potentially dangerous occupations such as flying or nuclear duties. Military psychiatrists also function as traditional psychiatric consultants assisting in evaluation and treatment of inpatients and outpatients in general hospitals.

Military psychiatrists may be called upon to aid civilian communities faced with disasters, as in the Gander-Newfoundland plane crash in December 1985. In the spring of 1989, military psychiatrists were consulted using a telemedicine space bridge to aid in the recovery of the Armenian earthquake and the Ufa (Russia) train disaster victims. Similarly, victims of hostage takings overseas may receive their first evaluations and treatment by military psychiatrists.

Military Psychiatrists as Educators

As educators, military psychiatrists are teachers and supervisors for professionals and nonprofessionals. Unit commanders, psychiatric technicians, and others are taught effective principles of primary and secondary prevention, including early identification of signs and symptoms of stress reactions, depression, suicidal risk, and substance abuse. Qualified and interested psychiatrists can serve as volunteer or full-time faculty at the Uniformed Services University of the Health Sciences (USUHS) School of Medicine, meeting the academic needs of 600 military medical students while pursuing clinical and basic science research.

Military Psychiatrists as Administrators

In the military, the administrator's role varies with his or her specific service, rank structure, and tenure, and with where he or she is stationed. More senior ranking and experienced psychiatrists may be commanders of mental health clinics, chiefs of clinical services in training hospitals, program directors of psychiatric residencies, or consultants to the Office of the Surgeon General. In these roles military psychiatrists function as administrators, consultants, and supervisors in making manpower decisions and developing policies and programs.

Career Issues

Career Options

A military psychiatrist's service career can begin as early as high school with involvement in the Reserve Officers' Training Corps (ROTC), followed by attendance at a civilian medical school via the Health Professionals Scholarship Program (HPSP) or at the Department of Defense (DOD) medical school, the USUHS School of Medicine. Residency training in the service may take place at military teaching hospitals.

Following residency, field tours as a general psychiatrist are encouraged, whether overseas or in the continental United States. Since the start of the all-volunteer armed forces, fully trained psychiatrists may also volunteer directly for service. A psychiatrist may pursue a career in direct clinical work, psychiatric consultation, academic psychiatry, research, or administration. There are also opportunities to work in the specialized areas of aerospace medicine, child and adolescent psychiatry, drug and alcohol abuse, and forensic psychiatry. Careers usually unfold based on the psychiatrist's talents and interests, the branch of service he or she is in, and service needs and opportunities. At present there are 345 active duty board-eligible or board-certified psychiatrists in the Army, Navy, and Air Force (personal communications with Army, Navy, and Air Force Consultants to the Surgeon General, November 1994).

Economics and Benefits of Military Psychiatry

Not all individuals find military life attractive or rewarding. If you want a life that is safe, uneventful, and predictable and prefer roots established in a single community with sameness in residence and daily experience, then it is unlikely that you will pursue the variety of missions and worldwide places of assignment offered with psychiatric practice in the military. The hallmark of a military career is its versatility and flexibility, its wide range of opportunities, and the membership it offers in a worldwide community and network of colleagues and friends.

A military psychiatrist's salary is based on rank, length of time in service, and medical specialty credentials (e.g., board certifications). Although military psychiatrists do not earn as much as their peers in private practice, they also do not have many of the financial burdens of private practice. Military psychiatry provides an alternative to the expensive administrative burdens of private practice by eliminating worries such as billing, diagnosis-related groups, malpractice insurance, third-party payers, and overhead costs. A complete range of specialists for consultation is also available to assist in assessment, consultation, and treatment and can be obtained without concern for medical insurance limits or patients' ability to pay.

In general, a military psychiatrist has 30 days of paid vacation annually, can attend one professional conference a year, can expect an excellent noncontributory retirement plan, and, when possible, has a choice of assignments through career planning.

Training

The Military Medical Corps provides training for many qualified physicians. In psychiatry, the task is not only to train future well-qualified, board-eligible general psychiatrists, but also to teach them the knowledge and skills necessary to treat the military community. Broad-based programs teach the knowledge and skills taught in civilian programs as well as military medical training and community psychiatry (Hales and Jones 1983). Teaching is based on primary prevention—reducing the incidence of problems in the military environment; secondary prevention—early identification and prompt treatment of psychiatric disorders; and tertiary prevention—managing psychiatrically ill patients to reduce chronicity and increase retention (Hales and Jones 1983; Hales et al. 1987).

At present, the military has nine approved residency programs and four child residency programs. There are also opportunities for postresidency training in administrative, consultation-liaison, and forensic psychiatry as well as psychoanalytic fellowships. There are no psychiatric hospitals within the military. Military training programs are conducted in major medical centers, usually in metropolitan areas. The military hospital system is the country's largest health maintenance organization, second only to the Veterans Administration system. It offers the complete spectrum of psychiatric services necessary for training psychiatrists and subspecialists.

Women and Minority Issues

As in any other professional or organizational structure, women in the military share similar dilemmas with other minority groups. The number of women in the services has increased in recent years and career opportunities have been expanded. Women and other minorities are actively recruited for the service academies as well as the Military Medical School at USUHS. At present, women make up 11.5% of the military population.

Career paths in military medicine are not closed to any individual. Diversity, equality, and opportunity are available to all. Professional challenges for women and minorities exist, as in the civilian community. Minority role models among faculties and administration may be few or absent. At times this leads to a feeling of alienation, distrust of leadership, a sense of self-isolation, or the wish to drop out. Even mentors knowledgeable about sociocultural variations are few. However, with time and an increase in military membership, those in the military, through networking, have been able to obtain the support and help to strengthen their identity as female or minority military officers and psychiatrists. Minority psychiatric residents and staff are increasing.

Women's special needs are being met through new policies such as the 6-week maternity leave. Although there is no specific family leave provision, up to 30 days can be taken from general leave time. Even military psychiatric training programs are flexible, allowing and offering electives and research time during the last trimester of pregnancy.

The military needs minority physicians with appropriate assertiveness and imagination to bring important perspective and skills to the care of the military community.

Ethical Considerations

Ethical issues in military psychiatry include the issue of "double agency"—that is, being in both the patient care role and the organizational physician role. Confidentiality and psychiatric labeling must be dealt with forthrightly to safeguard patients' rights and community safety.

Confidentiality. Military psychiatrists take care of the health, both physical and emotional, of active duty and retired service members and their families. As military officers, they must also advise commanders on medical issues that may affect accomplishment of a mission on which the nation's security may rest. Thus, in the military, active duty members have no direct right to confidentiality; however, neither do commanders have unrestricted access to patient records. Intimate details of a service member's life are not necessary to establish fitness for duty. In practice, military psychiatrists are afforded as much privacy in interactions with service members, and even more with their dependents and retirees, as are civilian psychiatrists in the age of third-party payers.

Stigma of psychiatric treatment. The problem of stigma associated with labeling exists in the military as in the civilian community. Military personnel may be reluctant to be seen by psychiatrists and receive a psychiatric diagnosis. Pilots, for example, frequently avoid medical and mental health care out of concern that their diagnoses and medications could mean temporary grounding. Many service members express concern that emotional problems may preclude promotions or lead to medical separation. Military psychiatrists are called upon to assess service members' suitability for duty in order to protect not only the individual but the unit and mission, just as civilian psychiatrists must protect the public from dangerous patients. Patients' irrational fears as well as legitimate concerns must be addressed forthrightly by military psychiatrists.

Military Psychiatry in the 1990s

Military psychiatry will encounter many new social and scientific issues in the 1990s. As the military faces downsizing, the practice of psychiatry confronts a greater challenge to maintain the missions of readiness, accessibility, quality of care, research, graduate medical education, and career development.

A recent change in policy, necessary to implement the DOD Homosexual Conduct Policy (Public Law 103-60, codified at

10 U.S.C. § 654 [1994]), is that a person's sexual orientation is a personal and private matter. It is not a bar to entry or to continued service unless manifested by homosexual conduct. Applicants for enlistment, appointment, or induction into the military will not be asked or required to reveal whether they are heterosexual, homosexual, or bisexual.

The concept of remedicalization of psychiatry is not controversial in the military because assessments and treatments have always used a strong biopsychosocial medical model. Military psychiatry must continue to be on the cutting edge of its scientific database, answering questions of psychiatric risk, illness prevention, and the problems of ever-changing military demographics. There is an ongoing commitment to scientific research in the areas of disasters, PTSD, AIDS, stress responses experienced in undersea and aerospace medicine, as well as others.

Conclusion

In this chapter, we have explored careers in military psychiatry. We have focused on defining the military psychiatrist's role as a community and consultation-liaison psychiatrist, describing the work setting and challenges inherent in treating and working with the military community. Economics, benefits, training opportunities, women's roles, and minority and ethical issues were also discussed. The practice of psychiatry in the military can be summed up as the practice of community psychiatry with diverse opportunities, good resources, and an organizational structure designed to provide worldwide delivery of care.

References

Belenky GL: Varieties of reaction and adaptation to combat experience. Bull Menninger Clin 1:64–79, 1987

Crocker LP: The Army Officer's Guide. Harrisburg, PA, Stockbridge Books, 1981

Hales RE, Jones FD: Teaching the principles of combat psychiatry to Army psychiatry residents. Milit Med 148:24–27, 1983

Hales RE, Borus JF, Privitera CF: Unique characteristics of Army psychiatry residency programs. Bull Menninger Clin 51:38–48, 1987

Menninger WW: Military psychiatry: learning from experience—introduction. Bull Menninger Clin 51:3–5, 1987

Ursano RJ: Military psychiatry: a triservice perspective (USAF Technical Report USAFSAM-TR-86-35). San Antonio, TX, USAF School of Aerospace Medicine, Brooks Air Force Base, January 1987

Ursano RJ, Holloway HC: Military psychiatry, in Comprehensive Textbook of Psychiatry/IV, 4th Edition, Vol 2. Edited by Kaplan H, Sadock B. Baltimore, MD, Williams & Wilkins, 1985, pp 1900–1910

Ursano RJ, Holloway HC, Jones DR, et al: Psychiatric care in the military community: family and military stressors. Hosp Community Psychiatry 40:1284–1289, 1989

Section II: Setting-Related Careers

Academic Psychiatry

CHAPTER FOURTEEN

Academic Psychiatry

Leah J. Dickstein, M.D.

Because all medical students and, of course, psychiatry residents rotate at different sites in their respective psychiatry departments and interact to varying degrees with a number of faculty, discussion of an academic psychiatry career at first glance might seem superfluous. However, unless one has worked closely with full-time faculty members, chances are slight that this career option is truly understood. Furthermore, a specialist in any of the areas covered in this book might be an academic psychiatrist.

The purpose of this chapter is threefold: to describe the scope of available academic opportunities; to define academic missions; and to outline benefits and problems of academic life, including unique issues for minority groups and for women as an underrepresented group.

Academic Opportunities

Practice in Psychiatric Subspecialties

As the 1990s—labeled the "decade of the brain"—progress toward the 21st century, opportunities in academic psychiatry continue to expand. There are 126 United States and 16 Canadian allopathic medical schools, and opportunities within each vary depending on the size and budget of the psychiatry department. In smaller departments, the type of services offered may be mostly general inpatient and outpatient adult, adolescent, and child services, plus consultation-liaison and emergency services. At the other end of the spectrum, larger departments may maintain a considerable variety of subspecialty divisions, clinics, services, and programs in addition to general psychiatry; for example:

- Alcohol and substance abuse
- Eating disorders
- Gender-specific programs (e.g., women's programs, men's units)
- Geriatric units
- Community and social psychiatry programs
- Day treatment programs
- Halfway and quarterway programs
- Anxiety and obsessive-compulsive disorders clinics
- Gender disorder and sexual dysfunction programs
- College programs
- Forensic units
- Behavioral psychiatry divisions, including cognitive and behavioral therapy units
- Pain clinics
- Sleep disorders units
- Family programs
- Group programs
- Acquired immunodeficiency syndrome sections as part of or separate from a neuropsychiatry unit
- Psychopharmacology units and clinics (e.g., clozapine clinics)
- Schizophrenia units
- Mood disorders units or clinics
- Personality and dissociative disorders units
- A psychoanalytic institute
- Arts and medicine divisions, including art, music, dance, and psychodrama programs
- Other innovative programs that include rheumatoid arthritis peer counselors and other emerging specialists who bring new therapies and skills to patient care and research protocols

Opportunities for further specialization in academic psychiatry include consultation-liaison services to just one unit (e.g., obstetrics-gynecology, surgery, oncology). Many academic departments also have Veterans Administration affiliations so that further special opportunities abound to work with veterans, with their significant others, and with the problems of posttraumatic stress disorder.

Administrative Responsibilities

Available opportunities. As part of these subjectively focused academic opportunities, faculty may also simultaneously seek or be assigned leadership responsibilities and experiences in these areas. On joining a certain faculty, a psychiatrist may be given the additional responsibility of becoming a clinic or program director; division, unit, or ward chief; or associate or assistant chief. Other administrative roles include director, assistant director, and associate director of medical student education or residency training, either for the entire department or for one hospital attached to the department. Obviously, every department administration includes a department chair (or head) as well as vice and associate chairs who are often responsible for certain areas (e.g., education, research, clinical services).

Acquiring administrative skills. Administrative responsibilities are assumed, perhaps without specific education or training, except if one has served as chief resident. Silver and Marcos (1989) delineated major factors involved in the evolution of the psychiatrist-executive who generally receives little administrative training during residency. An increasing number of faculty members who assume administrative roles also register for in-depth seminars, and others enroll in master's of business administration, master's of public health, and doctoral programs.

Silver and Marcos (1989) listed the following personality traits as helpful in administrators:

- The ability to create or focus and to concentrate on outcomes
- Good communication skills
- The ability to synthesize from theoretical and practical referents
- Persistence
- Self-direction
- Reliability and ability to capitalize on personal strengths
- Perseverance
- Creativity
- Initiative

Administrators are also more likely to be action oriented, possess good intuition and judgment, see problems as interrelated, and tolerate high degrees of ambiguity, novelty, and surprise (Silver and Marcos 1989). (See also discussion of administrative opportunities in Chapter 15.)

Joining academic societies, such as the Association for Academic Psychiatry, the Association of Directors of Medical Student Education in Psychiatry, or the American Association of Directors of Psychiatric Residency Training; reading these organizations' journals (e.g., *Academic Psychiatry*) and newsletters; and attending their meetings as well as the annual American Psychiatric Association (APA) meeting, with over 15,000 attendees, enable junior faculty to meet colleagues with similar interests, expertise, and wishes to network. In 5 very full days at the APA annual meeting, faculty can also avail themselves of lectures, discussion groups, research exhibits, and hallway consultations with world-famous researchers and clinicians who enjoy responding to junior faculty queries.

Committee Assignments

Assignments to committees such as admissions, curriculum, promotion and tenure, research, and even mundane ones like parking, to name the most recognizable, within the university and within the community as university liaison, are just a bare outline of possibilities (and probabilities) to which junior faculty can devote time and energy and begin to build careers. Committee work can enable newcomers to meet potential professional collaborators and friends and become more acquainted with the medical school, its environs and policies, and the university as a whole.

Private Practice

In addition to all of the above options and responsibilities, private practice of some degree is a further time commitment. In fact, an increasing number of full-time academics must "earn" (i.e., self-generate) their salaries by seeing patients privately because of department budget constraints. Often faculty are referred challenging patients who appear unresponsive to generally accepted treatments; faculty also serve as consultants to other external clinics, hospitals, centers, agencies, and national referral sources.

Academic Missions

Teaching and Supervising

Why do psychiatrists desire to work in academic settings? Most enjoy the opportunity and challenge of teaching students, residents, and other health trainees, and, of necessity, being themselves informed and conversant, not only about currently accepted diagnoses and treatment options, but about the frontiers of psychiatric knowledge and research. All physicians, and therefore psychiatrists, are, by definition, teachers (from the Latin derivative of the word "physician"). In the course of clinical practice, they teach patients and their families and significant others about patients' illnesses, treatment options, and protocols; they also teach their nursing and other professional staff.

However, medical school teaching is definitely different. Not to be overlooked is the almost paradoxical situation of junior faculty being assigned teaching responsibilities without being trained in medical teaching. It is fortunate that an increasing number of schools have offices of education with staff knowledgeable about the theory and reality of medical education. Conferences as well as journals are available from which neophytes can begin to learn and develop rational, proven teaching techniques. Beyond these formal intellectual learning options, junior faculty should be encouraged to invite senior faculty to observe and critique their efforts without fear of negative repercussions.

Teaching preclinical students usually occurs in large lecture halls or in small groups in conference rooms, on wards, and in patients' rooms. Effective lecturers do not read their lectures verbatim nor drone on endlessly or in unprepared fashion. Rather, accomplished and respected lecturers appropriately develop interest in their topics by devoting intensive time to careful preparation of handouts and useful, inoffensive (e.g., nonsexist or other biased) slides, and other audiovisual materials to enable students to absorb the concepts and facts clearly and usefully, rather than being challenged to simply memorize disconnected facts. Furthermore, preclinical lecturers, in core courses such as "Introduction to Psychiatry" and "Behavioral Science," must be able to maintain the interest of those students who have advanced college backgrounds in areas where most of their peers have only cursory knowledge.

Preclinical lecturers in psychiatry must also be able to withstand and contend with, without taking personal affront from, students' fears and lifelong stigma toward psychiatry, psychiatrists, and psychiatric illnesses. Academic psychiatrists, in their contacts with preclinical students, can affect the future general medical and psychiatric care of generations of patients by drawing students' attention to the actual capabilities of psychiatrists to treat genetically, biochemically, and environmentally based diseases in a scientific manner developed from a specific body of knowledge ranging from understanding the mind to psychoneuroimmunology, as would any physician in any other specialty. Preclinical teachers can also stimulate students' interests in research into unexplored areas, again as in all other medical specialties.

Preclinical lecturers in psychiatry also potentially influence all future physicians' attitudes toward their patients in the physician-patient nonverbal and verbal relationship. An often overlooked consequence of preclinical lecturing is the precious and unique opportunity to enable students to recognize vulnerabilities and problems within themselves simply by the lecturer's presentation of all topics, and especially presentations about particularly sensitive areas that young adults are likely to veer away from studying within themselves. Often, following a lecture, students with personal or family problems approach a respected teacher who appears to care about patients and their psychiatric illnesses because they sense that the teacher has an authentic interest in students and in helping others. These informal contacts can result in personal referral; what appears simply as a faculty member listening can, in reality, be a lifesaving act.

Teaching students who are rotating on psychiatry is also an exciting challenge, particularly because many are beginning to include and exclude future specialties as professional options as they complete rotations. Lectures to juniors, usually in small groups, entail clinical topics related to diagnosis and treatment. In addition, if lecturers have particular interests and feel students would benefit from hearing about them, lecturers can submit requests for lecture time to the department medical student education committee. For example, for the past 10 years I have taught a core lecture on "Gender Issues in Medical Practice" to juniors on psychiatry rotation. In this course, I cover sex role socialization, as well as different gender issues across the life cycle, including dependency, depression, child and spouse abuse, and suicide. Also, for the past 4 years I have taught a core lecture entitled "Behavioral Medicine" to juniors on psychiatry rotation.

In addition to lectures, faculty preside at conferences where students present patients with interesting and difficult problems for faculty response and recommendations.

Beyond student teaching and clinical supervision of junior students' care of patients, faculty also teach, supervise, and are responsible for residents' learning and patient care. Faculty teach seminars on

- Human development across the life cycle
- Psychopathology, including specific major psychiatric disorders, their diagnosis, and their treatment
- Theories of the mind
- Research
- Forensic issues
- Theories and techniques of psychotherapy
- Psychoanalysis
- Brief cognitive-behavioral therapies
- Dyadic, family, group therapies
- Current topics published in professional journals (journal club)

Faculty must make time to mentor residents and junior faculty. Faculty members supervise residents on clinical services and, in addition, generally serve as long-term psychotherapy supervisors for one or two residents throughout their residency.

Research

Some departments have separate research institutes. Most faculty have clinical responsibilities within general and specialized units and conduct research within their own units or in other units with colleagues. In addition to psychiatric faculty, departments include research and clinical psychologists, medical sociologists, and theologians who also conduct research while directing hospital chaplaincy training. (See Chapter 1 for details on the research arena.)

Although it may seem superfluous to mention research involvement and consequent publications as a prime responsibility for an academic psychiatrist, too frequently junior faculty assume that because of their clinical and even teaching responsibilities they can delay becoming involved in research and consequent publishing. They later realize that without having done such research, they will not meet the criteria and deadline for promotion and tenure, if tenure exists at their institution. This trauma can be avoided if department chairs assume appropriate responsibility to directly guide or oversee, and assign senior mentors to, junior faculty early in their careers.

Benefits and Difficulties in an Academic Career

Benefits

The material already outlined above should leave little doubt about the many varied opportunities that an academic career can offer. In addition to those mentioned above, academic psychiatrists can expect office expenses and billing to be assumed by the department. Night and weekend call are also rotated. Consultation with one's department peers, as well as with leading national academic researchers, clinicians, and teachers, can bring the cutting edge of research developments and consequent excellent patient care easily into one's office. Personal opportunities to present research at meetings locally and worldwide are stimulating rewards for perseverance beyond clinical competence for good patient care.

Problematic Issues

As in most academic medical careers, earning potential in academic psychiatry is less than in full-time clinical practice. However, with changes in reimbursement for patient care and in state budgets for medical school support, clinical faculty tracks have gained popularity. On a clinical track, faculty are expected to see patients and be available for on-site clinic and ward teaching. Research and consequent publication, although not requirements, may be pursued as well. Thus, clinical faculty tracks combine both clinical and faculty duties—the best of both worlds.

Junior faculty must be aware of and become informed about "academic politics" as part of the process to advancement. Although in recent years part-time academic appointments were available, economic constraints have curtailed such flexibility. Beyond devoting time and energy to teaching and clinical and administrative responsibilities, all junior faculty need mentors themselves.

Social Issues

Racial issues. Psychiatrists from racial minority populations remain underrepresented on academic psychiatry rosters and are definitely sought as potential faculty recruits. They serve not only as competent psychiatrists, but also as excellent role models for students, residents, and peer faculty in psychiatry and other departments, and clearly also as role models for patients, patients' families and significant others, staff, and all others with whom they come in contact. Sought after for committee work, at times to represent minority issues, they must make careful choices of ways they wish to spend their time without overcommitment.

Gender issues. As increasing numbers of women enter medicine, they also continue to specialize in psychiatry, as they always have. At present, women remain underrepresented at senior ranks in academia; there are only three women psychiatry department chairs in United States university programs and none in Canadian programs. Women continue to enter psychiatry, as do men, because of their interest in 1) the whole patient, 2) offering humanistic care, and 3) advances in neuroscience research and the cutting edge of pharmacological research and treatment issues, including unique differences and issues in these areas for women (Dickstein and Nadelson 1986). Myers (1982) wrote of the need for

> the encouragement and facilitation of female psychiatrists into academia to serve as role models for female (and male) trainees, to engage in topical research, to teach medical students and residents, and, most importantly, to supervise psychotherapy by *both* male and female residents. (p. 238)

Women faculty at the junior level too often either do not seek out mentors or find senior mentors less readily accessible than do their male peers (Penfold 1987). All faculty must become increasingly aware of gender issues, so that professional relationships at all levels are appropriately supportive and productive. Without ongoing discussion and experienced guidance by senior faculty about one's research interests, plans, activities, outcomes, papers, presentations, and the steps to reach publication, a successful long-term academic career is unlikely. Joint projects with faculty at one's own institution or with colleagues at other institutions are feasible, invigorating, and frequently fruitful.

In 1990 at the University of Louisville, I chaired a committee of residents and faculty that developed a resident parental leave policy to appropriately meet the needs of women and men trainees. This policy received full department support. Such policies should exist for faculty as well.

Issues for international medical graduates. The history and growth pre- and post-World War II of academic psychiatry are attributable in major aspects to internationally trained physicians who continue to seek careers in academic psychiatry in the United States and Canada but are often underrepresented. Beyond their individual abilities, these physicians bring cultural diversity to enrich everyone's education and, therefore, expertise in relating to all patients.

Conclusion

A career in academic psychiatry offers a multiplicity of opportunities, challenges, variety and breadth of potential satisfaction in patient care, research, teaching, administration, collegiality, and professional education and development that, with proactive planning and timely mentoring, are unquestionably worth the enormous efforts needed to become and remain a successful academician.

References

Dickstein LJ, Nadelson CC: Women Physicians in Leadership Roles. Washington, DC, American Psychiatric Press, 1986

Myers MF: The professional woman as patient: a review and an appeal. Can J Psychiatry 27:236–240, 1982

Penfold SP: Women in academic psychiatry in Canada. Can J Psychiatry 32:660–665, 1987

Silver MA, Marcos LR: The making of the psychiatrist-executive. Am J Psychiatry 146:29–34, 1989

Section III: Administrative Psychiatry

CHAPTER FIFTEEN

Administrative Psychiatry

Carolyn B. Robinowitz, M.D.

Perceptions of Administration by Psychiatrists

Studies have estimated that 10% of psychiatrists' work time is spent in administration (Fenton 1987), with increasing demands for administrative skills for those working in service delivery settings, with other professionals involved in patient care, and as team leaders in inpatient units, ambulatory care settings, community mental health programs, academic psychiatry departments, and other treatment and administrative settings. Clinical psychiatrists—with their knowledge of individual and group psychodynamics—often are in a good position to work through the intricacies of multifactorial management systems and may become administrators of treatment teams, clinical care settings, university departments, or county or state mental health programs.

The following descriptions indicate the arenas in which psychiatrists formally—and informally—exercise administrative skills:

- *Psychiatrists in hospitals* provide leadership, interact with groups, plan and monitor patients' treatment, and interface with other health and mental health professionals, social systems, and legal networks, providing direct and indirect consultation to a wide panoply of caregivers.
- The *clinician in practice* must deal with external administrative forces related to third-party reimbursement, managed care, and financial systems; with legal issues; and with generic treatment systems.
- A *university department chairperson* spends a considerable amount of time in fund-raising and "union arbitrating" while administering or delegating responsibility in a complex system that provides

education at many levels, undertakes research, and provides for clinical care.
- A *public psychiatrist* must demonstrate agility and sophistication in epidemiology, planning, budgeting, legal issues, working with legislators and government representatives, and dealing with advocacy groups and the media.
- *Rural psychiatrists* must work well with public health nurses, voluntary human service agencies, police and sheriffs, clergy, general hospital administrators, and other health and mental health clinicians and program planners. Comprehensive care requires considerable familiarity with disparate cultural and geographic settings and the often fragmented transportation systems connecting them, finances of care delivery, as well as the specific clinical issues affecting the patients.
- The *manager of one or more inpatient or partial hospitalization services* must develop, monitor, and evaluate treatment approaches; work with staff within treatment settings to provide first-rate care; and integrate education and research programs with service needs. Utilizing a public health approach for prevention, as well as early intervention, and developing community-based care systems, the administrator may take charge of a unit within a county or state health department.
- *Administrators in charge of clinical research centers* must intermingle research interests with those of clinical care; they may be engaged in developing school or hospital-based consultation programs to deal with children at risk; they may be working within medical specialty organizations dealing with issues of mental health policy or working with federal and local governments to ensure availability of funding and resources for the prevention and treatment of mental disorders.

Psychiatrists in these diverse settings all need administrative skills. Experts agree that there is a critical shortage of trained, experienced psychiatrist-administrators. They are needed at all levels of responsibility to cope with the increasing regulation of cost and quality of care and thus to help shape mental health policies that determine the delivery of psychiatric care.

Characteristics of an Effective Administrator

The functions of "clinician-executives" (Greenblatt and Rose 1977; Levinson and Klerman 1967, 1973) are stimulating and challenging. These psychiatrists often speak of their careers as the best of both worlds—being able to maintain a clinical knowledge base while translating clinical skills into more systematic work. Administrators dealing with groups and systems must understand roots of interpersonal tension, authority, and power structures within organizations. One of the joys of good administration is the major positive impact an administrator can have on education, research, and patient care. Further, because many administrative opportunities are in the public sector, psychiatrist-administrators can gain great satisfaction from working to improve care in communities and thus have an impact on underserved groups. Serving as educators, administrators promote interest in the area, as well as define and enhance the knowledge base through modeling, demonstration, and supervision, and affect the administrative ability and performance of clinicians, and thus, clinical care.

Effective administrators work at a brisk and engaging pace often characterized by brevity, variety, and discontinuity (Hinkle and Burns 1978; Silver and Marcos 1989). Tolerating and even thriving on high degrees of ambiguity and novelty, acting while thinking, and seeing problems as interrelated, they are strongly action oriented and process information linking the organization with its environment. This blend of intuition and rational judgment also is the mark of a good clinician and underscores the connection between the clinical and administrative areas.

Added to the core skill and identity of a clinical psychiatrist is the intellectual understanding of administrative principles and development of technical managerial skills in implementing these principles (Bennis and Nanus 1985), including the ability to create a focus and to concentrate on outcomes, good communication skills, and the ability to synthesize from the theoretical to the practical. Personal qualities include initiative and self-direction, persistence, motivation, creativity, reliability, and the ability to capitalize on personal strengths.

Administrators must build on their clinical knowledge to learn how to deal with issues in groups, as well as in individual interactions; prioritize and allocate often scarce resources; and find ways to solve problems that end up with a *win-win approach* (i.e., an approach in which both sides feel they have accomplished much). Understanding motivation is essential for successful negotiating and decision making. It is important that a psychiatrist-administrator avoid becoming a therapist for the staff members, unit, or system. Although sick systems deserve attention and individual behaviors must be considered, a wise administrator will consider them within an organizational structural framework rather than as a clinician dealing with individual pathology. The administrator should be aware of the importance of affect and unresolved issues even to mental health professionals and recognize that all staff members have some imperfections and limits. At the same time, psychodynamic or diagnostic interpretations do not get the work done. Thus, the challenge becomes dealing with individual needs in the context of the work to be done.

Education and Training

There is a dearth of formal educational or training experiences in administration during psychiatry residency (Borus 1983; Bucher 1965; Sherwood et al. 1986; Taintor and Robinowitz 1987; Talbott and Sachs 1982). Many psychiatrists have commented that they entered administrative positions by chance or through luck and learned administration on the job. This learning by doing can be a hit-or-miss phenomenon, unless there is a degree of cognitive organization to what is essentially an experiential process. Most residency training programs provide some didactic training through seminars, but organized education in this area is limited.

Some residency programs offer seminars on aspects of administration, including topics such as legal issues, group dynamics, and leadership functions. There are few, if any, formal opportunities to learn about planning, financing and health economics, and systems design and analysis as part of residency experience. Some programs have a more extensive curriculum in administration, with required as well as elective courses that combine theoretical and experiential work. (For information about such opportunities, the *American Psychiatric Association Directory of Psychiatry Residency Programs* contains data about required and elective training.)

Hands-on administrative experience most likely occurs within the last 2 years of residency, during which the resident may serve as a chief resident on an inpatient unit or ambulatory service. Being a chief resident is an important growth experience, conveying both clinical knowledge and skills and administrative-managerial complexities. Some programs offer a chief residency lasting from a few months to a year for all or most senior residents, allowing them to be involved in a specific area or setting; others reserve the experience for one or two gifted leaders who may be responsible for many of the administrative and managerial decisions regarding residents' work loads, on-call schedules, patient assignments (working in conjunction with educational faculty), and departmental function. They may also provide (and receive) various forms of supervision related to organizational structure, staff function, and so on (Grant et al. 1974; Looney et al. 1975; Sherman 1972).

There also are yearlong postresidency fellowships that emphasize administrative theory, program planning, personnel and human resources deployment, legal and ethical issues, financial planning, and health economics, as well as care management and evaluation (Feldman 1974).

Other educational opportunities can be gained through course work in schools of business administration, public health, public administration, or even law. Whereas such schools offer a formal educational program—with specific entry requirements leading to a master's or doctoral degree—individual courses in public health, health policy management, finances, planning, and so forth can also be extremely helpful for the neophyte administrator. Each approach focuses on a different area, but all provide some of the knowledge base needed for administration. Most programs in business administration and public administration tend to be designed for nonclinicians, often providing more information about business and political systems than may be needed (although there are a few graduate programs that focus on business administration in health care delivery systems). Similarly, public health programs can offer electives or concentrations in mental health, and clinicians can take courses in psychiatry and the law. Whereas all of these types of programs can be useful, administrative psychiatry fellowships focus primarily on what can be described as the skills of the clinician-executive, combining a cognitive knowledge base with specific hands-on administrative-clinical experience in the mental health setting.

Accreditation of Administrative Psychiatry as a Specialty

Currently there is no formal accreditation of postresidency programs in administrative psychiatry; such accreditation is offered in child psychiatry, geriatric psychiatry, and addiction psychiatry. The American Board of Psychiatry and Neurology (ABPN) offers certificates of added qualification in geriatric psychiatry, addiction psychiatry, and forensic psychiatry.

It is possible, however, for individual psychiatrists to document and demonstrate their qualifications. Since 1953, the American Psychiatric Association (APA) has offered certification in administrative psychiatry, a certificate developed to emphasize the field as a specialized area of medical practice as well as to recognize and support psychiatric hospital directors. About 350 psychiatrists currently hold this certificate. To be eligible, applicants must first be certified in psychiatry by the ABPN and have had a minimum of 3 years' experience in a significant administrative role in a psychiatric program or at least 1 year's formal training and education postresidency in administration or a related field. The certification process consists of a written and oral examination, with the former component testing overall knowledge and the latter component testing skill in knowledge application and problem solving, meshing practical and clinical needs with theory (Foley 1971).

Skills Needed to Be Certified in Administrative Psychiatry

Although specific details of curriculum content vary from program to program, the following elements, addressed in the APA's examination, are the foundation for theoretical and practical knowledge and should be part of every postresidency training program (American Psychiatric Association 1993). *Administration,* broadly defined, includes the following:

- Authority and responsibility
- Management
- Personnel administration (including labor-management relations)
- Staff development and continuing education
- Organizational behavior
- Problem solving
- Decision making
- Program planning and evaluation
- Performance evaluation

Knowledge about *fiscal management* should include roles and functions of the financial manager within mental health organizations, accounting practices and budgeting in mental health systems, methods and mechanisms for financing mental health care (including the financial structure and organization of mental health facilities), role of funding sources, management, and accountability.

The psychiatric administrator should be cognizant of *legal and ethical issues,* including commitment procedures and rights, treatment rights and informed consent, other civil rights, confidentiality and privilege, record keeping, disclosure and access, ethical values, and the responsibilities of the psychiatrist.

In addition, there are specific administrative aspects to psychiatric care management that include both clinical and nonclinical issues, such as the following:

- Program design and implementation
- Interactions with other health and human services providers, consumers, government, and political, fiscal, and community bodies
- Accreditation
- Medical record keeping
- Program evaluation
- Utilization review and quality assurance

- Therapeutic milieu
- Programs for special groups, such as children, elderly individuals, multiply handicapped individuals, those who abuse substances, and those involved with the criminal justice system
- Interdisciplinary service delivery
- Epidemiology
- Public and community health concepts

Because *good clinical skills* are vital to administrative psychiatry, experience in administration should not be gained at the expense of basic clinical development or as a way to avoid the stresses of direct clinical care. A good residency with appropriate breadth and depth of experiences is the best preparation for an administrative career. One must be highly cognizant of clinical issues in diagnosis and treatment as well as prevention.

The clinician's understanding of groups' and the community's needs must be based on knowledge and skill in dealing with individuals. An elective or chief residency will provide initial exposure, but, in this day and age of subspecialization, it is reasonable to expect the clinician-executive to obtain additional formal learning experiences on a full- or part-time basis in a variety of schools and settings, combined with a practicum that encourages skill development and mastery. In addition, the practicum should provide exposure to other clinician-executives who can serve as advisers and role models as well as demonstrate positive attitudes about such work. This meshing with a senior and respected leader is especially important, as most of the mentors and admired leaders during residency are clinicians and researchers, who may not demonstrate interest or skill in administration (Hunt and Michael 1983; Ochberg et al. 1986). Further, many of the administrators observed during training may be nonmedical or nonclinical in background and experience, thus reinforcing the notion of administrators as nonclinical bureaucrats. Given the paucity of formal supervised educational experiences in administration and the need to develop more clinical and experiential skills as an administrator, closely supervised practicum work with a psychiatrist mentor is a vital aspect of professional development.

Experience in *research* is important, not only for its impact on critical thinking, but as an opportunity to develop an understanding of the process of problem identification, hypothesis formation, and test data gathering and analysis within the context of an administrative system. An administrator with experience in and understanding of research is more likely to be supportive of ongoing research, which adds to the knowledge base of the field and promotes better clinical care. Administrators who encourage or participate in research also enrich their own career development as well as enhance their understanding.

Formal Course Work for Administrative Psychiatry

There are independently sponsored, brief courses on topics related to the content of the certifying examination in administrative psychiatry. Two related organizations provide continuing education in administration: the American College of Mental Health Administration and the American Association of Psychiatric Administrators. Groups such as the American Society of Association Executives, the American Association of Medical Society Executives, and the American College of Physician Executives also offer brief consultation and education. Involvement in the community of administrators provides enrichment. The young administrator should attend meetings to learn about new approaches and discoveries and to compare experiences and programs, as well as to make personal connections with leaders and colleagues.

Issues for Special Populations

Administrative careers attract a broad range of psychiatrists. Women and minority psychiatrists must cope with issues related to their minority status as well as the basic needs of their positions. International medical graduates (IMGs) who often work in the public sector face additional problems (Kessler et al. 1982; Robinowitz et al. 1981).

Traditionally, leaders in psychiatry as in other areas of medicine have been white males. Women and psychiatrists from other minority groups thus have to confront unmet expectations and stereotypes. They also must face the implications of both affirmative action and "glass ceilings." There may be overt or covert resistance to being supervised by a woman or a member of a minority population; search committees or senior administrators may have "old boy" networks or resist choosing women or minority members who do not "fit in" or who represent a shift in perspective. Women and minorities may experience less mentoring than their majority colleagues.

Nonetheless, women, those from minority populations, and IMGs are needed in administrative positions. Their personal and professional experiences as nonmajority members may be helpful in sensitizing them to issues of cultural diversity and transcultural differences in illness and health service delivery as well as in avoiding the overpersonalization that can come with facing racism or sexism in the workplace. Leaders in the field are working to expand not only entry-level opportunities for psychiatrists from these groups, but also opportunities for advancement into positions with increased authority as well as responsibility.

Benefits of an Administrative Psychiatric Career

Administration can be a good field for those who want more flexible work settings and hours. Administrative positions usually are salaried and often take place in a structured setting with less weekend, emergency, and on-call time demands than more intensive clinical work. Administrators may work full- or part-time and may combine their administrative work with more traditional clinical duties. Administration is generally not a highly paid area, but there is no overhead or expense associated with practice, and in many communities, net income is competitive with that in private practice.

Conclusion

Psychiatric administration covers a wide and exciting array of career opportunities. Demand for psychiatric administrators exists throughout the country in multiple settings, with ongoing opportunities for intellectual stimulation and growth. Clinician-executives have a strong sense of impact and accomplishment and, despite obstacles and frustration, voice much career satisfaction.

References

American Psychiatric Association, Committee on Administrative Psychiatry: Information Bulletin for Applicants, 12th Edition. Washington, DC, American Psychiatric Association, 1993

Bennis W, Nanus B: Leaders: The Strategies for Taking Charge. New York, Harper & Row, 1985

Borus JF: Teaching residents the administrative aspects of psychiatric practice. Am J Psychiatry 140:444–448, 1983

Bucher R: The psychiatric residency and professional socialization. J Health Soc Behav 6:197–206, 1965

Feldman S: Educating the future mental health executive: a graduate curriculum. Administration in Mental Health 3:74–85, 1974

Fenton WS: The professional activities of psychiatrists, in The Nation's Psychiatrists. Edited by Koran LM. Washington, DC, American Psychiatric Association, 1987, pp 77–95

Foley AR: Certification and training in administrative psychiatry. Hosp Community Psychiatry 22:69–73, 1971

Grant I, Dorus W, McGlashan T, et al: The chief resident in psychiatry. Arch Gen Psychiatry 30:503–507, 1974

Greenblatt M, Rose S: Illustrious psychiatric administrators. Am J Psychiatry 134:626–630, 1977

Hinkle A, Burns M: The clinician-executive: a review. Administration in Mental Health 6:3–21, 1978

Hunt DM, Michael G: Mentorship: a career training and development tool. Academy of Management Review 8:475–485, 1983

Kessler MD, Hellekson EC, Wilder JF: The psychiatric chief resident: does gender make a difference? Am J Psychiatry 139:1610–1613, 1982

Levinson DJ, Klerman GL: The clinician-executive: some problematic issues for the psychiatrist in mental health organizations. Psychiatry 30:3–15, 1967

Levinson DJ, Klerman GL: The clinician-executive revisited. Administration in Mental Health 1:64–67, 1973

Looney J, Engelberg S, Gode R, et al: The psychiatric chief residency: a preliminary training experience in administrative process. Am J Psychiatry 132:729–733, 1975

Ochberg RL, Tischler GL, Schulberg HC: Mentoring relationships in the careers of mental health administrators. Hosp Community Psychiatry 37:939–941, 1986

Robinowitz C, Nadelson C, Notman M: Women in academic psychiatry: politics and progress. Am J Psychiatry 138:1357–1361, 1981

Sherman R: The psychiatric chief resident. Journal of Medical Education 47:277–280, 1972

Sherwood E, Greenblatt M, Pasnau R: Psychiatric residency, role models, and leadership. Am J Psychiatry 143:764–767, 1986

Silver MA, Marcos LR: The making of the psychiatrist-executive. Am J Psychiatry 146:29–34, 1989

Taintor Z, Robinowitz CB: The Education and Professional Qualification of Psychiatrists. Washington, DC, American Psychiatric Association, 1987

Talbott JA, Sachs M: Teaching psychiatric administration to senior residents. Administration in Mental Health 9:281–288, 1982

Section IV:
Practice by Specialty Area

Focus on Unique Populations

CHAPTER SIXTEEN

Child Psychiatry

Helen R. Beiser, M.D.
Benjamin Garber, M.D.

History

Board certification in child psychiatry began in 1959, although the term *child psychiatry* was first used in 1935 by Kanner (1935) in his textbook of the same name. Only in this century have children been perceived as having special emotional needs that must be served by specially trained professionals. In 1899, the first juvenile court was established in Chicago, Illinois, in recognition that juvenile delinquents required different handling than adult criminals. In 1909, William Healy established a clinic in conjunction with a court (Healy 1915). He later founded Boston's Judge Baker Clinic; his original Chicago clinic became the statewide Institute for Juvenile Research (Beiser 1966). Through the auspices of the Commonwealth Fund, child guidance clinics modeled on these court clinics became widespread.

A parallel French development was the psychological testing of mentally retarded individuals (Binet and Simon 1916), widened with the use of tests for different populations, often in child guidance clinics.

Physicians with a special interest in children gradually formed a specialty—pediatrics—which achieved board certification in 1933. Although this certification brought a more biological orientation to children's care, pediatricians were also aware of psychological aspects of childhood behavior. Child psychiatry has been returning to its biological roots, especially with advances in the neurosciences. Child psychiatrists and pediatricians find it useful to work together in many complicated situations, as in the care of severely compromised infants and their families.

Another important root of child psychiatry is psychoanalysis. Some American psychiatrists traveled to Vienna in the 1920s and 1930s to study with Anna Freud and other analysts and became interested in the application of analytic principles to child therapy and child rearing. Aichhorn's work in Vienna (1925/1935) on delinquency was a connection to the American interest in juvenile delinquency. Psychoanalysis also focused on parent-child interactions as causative of emotional conflicts, and increased psychiatrists' understanding of adult patients in light of their patients' childhood experiences.

The official professional identity of child psychiatry crystallized in the post–World War II ferment of the 1950s, with formulation of criteria for training centers, individual training, and finally, board certification. Although child psychiatrists worked comfortably with other disciplines (e.g., social workers, psychologists), their medical background gave them a special identity and resulted in the formation of the American Academy of Child Psychiatry in 1953 (changed to the American Academy of Child and Adolescent Psychiatry [AACAP] in 1988). Today many child psychiatrists belong to both the AACAP and the multidisciplinary American Orthopsychiatric Association, established in 1925.

The Scope of Child Psychiatry

Child psychiatry's multiple origins provide for wide variation in professional practice, with room to adapt to children's changing needs, including those of children raised in single-parent households, cross-racial marriages, and divorced and adoptive families. Other problems child psychiatrists must deal with are those related to the greater cultural variation following the influx of many immigrant groups (e.g., resistance to acceptance of English as the common language) and greater social tolerance for early sexual activity. Improved medical treatment has produced more chronically disabled children, has spawned issues relating to organ transplants, and even has increased the possibility of drug use. Acquired immunodeficiency syndrome (AIDS) is becoming more common in teenagers and in infants of intravenous-drug–abusing mothers, bringing with it its own problems for children. In addition to these newer areas of work, ordinary childhood problems remain (e.g., those related to family and peer relationships, reactions to intercurrent illnesses, learning disabilities, poor impulse control from many causes, severe organic incapacities, and mental illness of a genetic nature).

Because the entire family's functioning is so important for the health of the child, some psychiatrists specialize in family therapy, treating parents and other relatives, such as grandparents and siblings. Work with parents is different from ordinary adult psychiatric therapy because the primary focus in family therapy is to facilitate the child's healing or growth.

Work Skills

Certain skills are essential for child psychiatrists, regardless of the setting in which they work (Chess and Hassibi 1978). Gathering data directly from children is the key skill and requires knowing developmental norms and how children communicate at different ages, along with the ability to interpret play, drawings, games, and other forms of communication suitable to a child's developmental level. The ability to evaluate a child's problem also requires information to be gathered from significant persons in the child's environment: the parents, other family members, schoolteachers, physicians, psychologists, social workers, and courts. It is not uncommon to find that a child appears quite different to each of these professionals. Intelligence tests, tests of neurological status, and general health may all be important. Integration of all of these observations into a diagnostic understanding of the child and his or her problem is one of the greatest challenges and satisfactions of the field.

After an evaluation, a treatment plan (Chess and Hassibi 1978) must be instituted. This may vary from suggestions to parents for handling difficult behavior differently to removal of a child from a chaotic home. Treatment may be focused directly on the child and/or indirectly, through suggesting changes in the home or school. Some psychiatric conditions respond well to medication (amphetamines have long been used for organic hyperactivity, but now drugs are available for panic, obsessive-compulsive, and bipolar disorders). Psychotherapy, either alone or in conjunction with medication, for the child, the parental figures, or both, is the most common intervention, whether symptom directed as in behavior modification or personality directed as in classical psychoanalysis. Some combination of treatment approaches is usual. Most child psychiatrists develop a preference for using just a few of the available treatment modalities but should be aware of others and recommend the most appropriate.

Work Settings

Most child psychiatrists work in private offices with children and families who seek help as outpatients. All the same skills are used also in clinic or group practice, and in hospitals where child psychiatrists have ongoing responsibility for patients' treatment. Communicating with third-party payers is increasingly necessary. If a child psychiatrist is salaried, he or she has a responsibility to the institution-employer; it is also important that the institution and the psychiatrist have the same concern for the child's welfare. Specific salaried job settings that are frequently advertised include pediatric wards, psychiatric hospitals, institutions for the mentally retarded, institutions for juvenile delinquents, long-term residential centers for youngsters with chronic character disorders, and academic positions in medical schools. Psychiatric consultation may be desired by school systems or by social agencies. Work with courts has become more diversified and includes clinics to aid courts with diagnosis and treatment planning for delinquents, diagnosis of child abuse, and determination of custody and visitation within the context of divorce cases.

Another mode of indirect child psychiatric treatment is through consultation-liaison with other professionals, including physicians who carry primary responsibility for the child's care. As a skill in its own right, consultation should be added to the skills of direct evaluation and treatment. School consultants assist school psychologists, social workers, and teachers in understanding the problems children present in school. Psychiatric consultants to social agencies assist social workers who deal with children whose families are disrupted and need auxiliary families. A new area of consultation-liaison psychiatry is helping in the care of the seriously compromised infant, especially in preparing the family for the necessary long-term care.

Training Requirements

With the broadening scope of child psychiatry, the special requirements for certification that have been approved by the Accreditation Council for Graduate Medical Education have grown more elaborate with each revision. Under the recent trend for psychiatry to return to its biological roots (Detre 1987), there has been an increased emphasis on the study of the neurobiological aspects of childhood and adolescence.

Three years of general psychiatry followed by 2 years of child psychiatry fellowship is the sequence developed for those seeking board certification in child psychiatry as a subspecialty of psychiatry. Various other arrangements may be approved, such as altering the sequence, or substituting clinical psychology, developmental pediatrics, or pharmacology for trainees who wish to enter research or academic careers. There is also an experimental triple board program at six selected training centers for those wishing certification in pediatrics, general, and child psychiatry. This program consists of 2 years of general pediatrics and 3 years of adult, adolescent, and child psychiatry, which allows the psychiatrist to complete training in these areas 1 year earlier than if the traditional training programs for each specialty had been followed.

A survey of training programs (Schowalter 1984) revealed that outpatient work, consultation with pediatricians, knowledge of psychopharmacology, and involvement in mandatory research were deemed essential skills to be learned. In training, the team concept remains, but the team members have increased in number and are more varied than in the past (i.e., they include professionals with other skills such as the expressive therapies, chaplain trainees, and those knowledgeable about behavioral medicine).

Research

Exploration of the epidemiology and outcome of various treatments for a multitude of clinical problems, and increasing knowledge in the basic biology of many conditions, provides unique research opportunities for child psychiatrists. Consultation may be related to individual cases or may be more formal and didactic. Consultants and teachers should be most aware of those problems requiring research, such as child abuse, teenage pregnancy, adolescent drug abuse, effects of various kinds of family disruption, possible neurobiological bases of many disorders, and the effectiveness of various types of treatment, including pharmacological treatment.

Economics

Of all the medical specialties, child psychiatry has the most pressing need for more psychiatrists. According to a 1983 AACAP report, "Child Psychiatry: A Plan for the Coming Decades," there were about 3,000 child psychiatrists in the United States in 1980, and the projected need was for a threefold increase by 1990. Although there has been an increase, it has not been of that magnitude, as demands outstrip training capacities.

According to the AACAP report, in 1983 the typical child psychiatrist was in solo practice in a city of less than 500,000 people, working mostly with outpatients, about half of whom were children and adolescents. The most common treatment modality was individual psychotherapy for an average of 49 weeks, with patients seen once or twice a week. The most common diagnoses were anxiety, conduct, and attention-deficit disorders.

Although the proportion of the population under age 18 years is declining, the number of disturbed children seems to be increasing for reasons that are unclear. One cause could be the disruption families are now experiencing. At the same time, there is declining support for special services in schools because of financial constraints, but a greater awareness of the need for psychiatric help in legal decisions regarding delinquency, child abuse, child custody, adoption, and foster care.

Child psychiatric services have increased in private clinics, mental health centers, university clinics, and especially in hospitals for adolescents (Jemerin and Philips 1988; Rafferty 1988). Often the treatment a child receives, and from whom, is not directly related to the nature of the child's need. The most economically lucrative area of practice today is the psychiatric hospitalization of adolescents, but, given questions regarding the appropriateness and cost-effectiveness of this very expensive treatment, its future is questionable.

Whereas in a general sense child psychiatric practice is thriving, there are several significant problems in the field. One is the lack of an adequate range of facilities for severely disturbed children and adolescents, especially for long-term care. Another problem, especially in the outpatient area, is competition from nonmedical therapists. The latter are usually somewhat less expensive than psychiatrists and carry less stigma for many parents. Outcome research would be useful to see if an apparently more expensive intervention does indeed have superior results.

Despite these problems, most child psychiatrists seem satisfied and happy with their work. Even if salaried physicians eventually replace the solo practitioner, opportunities in terms of geographic location and type of work are immense.

Special Legal Issues

Because an increasing number of children are involved in legal proceedings, no child psychiatrists currently practicing can remain aloof from the legal establishment (Benedek 1986; Chess and Hassibi 1978). In fact, many have joined general psychiatrists in setting up the specialty of forensic psychiatry. Even neophyte child psychiatrists may need to evaluate—and possibly treat—children suspected of being abused or children who are in the midst of a custody battle. Work with pediatricians or protective service workers may be necessary. Child psychiatrists must keep abreast of local laws regarding mandatory reporting of possible abuse and must know who has the legal rights to permit interviewing of the child.

The child psychiatrist asked to serve as an expert witness must provide an assessment of the child's emotional and intellectual status, outline the child's needs accordingly, and assist the court in weighing the influence of various organic and environmental factors. In custody decisions, it is preferable for the psychiatrist to be invited to participate by a judge or by a court-appointed lawyer for the child, rather than by the lawyer of one of the parents, in order to avoid the expectation of taking one parent's side, which is not necessarily for the child's benefit. Perhaps the most difficult custody decision the court has to make occurs when both parents have serious psychopathology. Here the child psychiatrist's expertise in separating parenting functions from more global psychopathology can be of great value.

Child psychiatrists may advise a court on the most appropriate handling of individual delinquents to help such youths function more adequately in society. Children may be exposed to extremely traumatic events and be asked to testify about them in court—a process that highlights the differences between the legal and the medical approaches. Child psychiatrists may not always be able to protect children from repeated cross-examinations, nor their families from the stresses of the legal procedures.

Two areas of the legal system to be avoided by child psychiatrists are malpractice suits and hearings on ethical violations. Although psychiatric malpractice suits are not common compared with those of many medical specialties, they do occur and usually involve perceived damages suffered by a patient while under care. Ethical violations are more common than malpractice suits; the tendency for children to seek physical contact with their therapist requires tactful handling by the therapist and caution about entering the gray area of perceived sexual abuse. Child psychiatrists must be aware of their state laws regarding medical practice and of the various ethical codes of the professional societies to which they belong. AACAP has devised a code of ethics tailored to clinical issues specific to this field.

Special Opportunities and Problems

Potential child psychiatrists should enjoy being with children, even when those children are angry or withdrawn and not very likable. This general professional ease with children seems to differentiate child from adult psychiatrists and presents a challenge, requiring real respect for children as individuals. Most children are unwilling patients, and it is hard to help them see themselves as needing help. Child psychiatrists must also have empathy for parents and other adults in the child's life in order not to fail the child in the long run.

Another challenge in working with children and adolescents is to get parents to agree to continuation of treatment for their child or to have adolescents agree to continue as long as the therapist feels treatment is desirable.

Children's tendency to communicate through action and express anger through destructive behavior can become another problem for the child psychiatrist who is growing older or has developed a physical disability.

One disadvantage of child psychiatry is its low status in medicine, in which anything relating to children tends to be denigrated, especially if play and games are used to communicate. It is significant that the AACAP was the last organization representing a board-certified specialty to gain a seat in the American Medical Association House of Delegates.

It is important for medical specialists to belong to a number of medical organizations, but there is a special camaraderie within the AACAP, with less of the competitiveness that mars some professional organizations.

A major pleasure of child psychiatry is the opportunity to see children change in response to treatment as well as through the natural process of maturation. Some patients who enter treatment as children are followed into adulthood; young adults may call or write former therapists to report on successes or to ask advice about current problems or decisions. Insight into the childhood of adult patients enriches the psychotherapy of adults.

Child psychiatry can provide minority groups and women with special opportunities. A number of African-American psychiatrists have done important work improving educational and medical services for economically disadvantaged families and minority families and their children. They are also important role models for disadvantaged minority children. Psychiatrists who come from backgrounds similar to their patients' and/or speak their language can best help special groups, such as children of migrant workers or illegal immigrants. It is, however, not always desirable for either patients or psychiatrists to match patients and psychiatrists of the same culture.

Women have a very distinct role in child psychiatry, possibly because they may relate to young children more naturally than do most men.

For patients who have grown up fearing their father, a woman may be the therapist of choice, at least at first. Mothers often feel that a woman is more understanding of their particular problems than a man. Women as supervisors of individual psychotherapy are usually well accepted by men and women students. Rather than needing to battle prejudice, women, particularly as clinicians, are seen as having distinctive value in the field of child psychiatry, though they may at times face special negative mother transferences from patients or from students. As teachers and administrators, women child psychiatrists face the same problems they face in any other medical field.

In summary, for physicians who enjoy and are curious about children and their problems and development, and who can be comfortable dealing with the often many adults in the child's environment, child psychiatry can be an enjoyable and satisfying profession.

References

Aichhorn A: Wayward Youth (English translation). New York, Viking Press, 1935 (original German edition published in 1925)

American Academy of Child and Adolescent Psychiatry: Child psychiatry: a plan for the coming decades. Washington, DC, American Academy of Child and Adolescent Psychiatry, 1983

Beiser HR: Fifty-seven years of child guidance: the experience of the Institute for Juvenile Research. Excerpta Medica International Congress Series 150, Proceedings of the Fourth World Congress of Psychiatry, 1966

Benedek E: Forensic child psychiatry. Bull Am Acad Psychiatry Law 14:295–300, 1986

Binet A, Simon T: The Development of Intelligence in Children. Baltimore, MD, Williams & Wilkins, 1916

Chess S, Hassibi M, eds: Principles and Practice of Child Psychiatry. New York, Plenum Press, 1978 (Assessment, pp 148–198, Treatment, pp 391–426, Law, pp 441–456)

Detre T: The future of psychiatry. Am J Psychiatry 144:621–626, 1987

Healy W: The Individual Delinquent. Boston, MA, Little, Brown, 1915

Jemerin J, Philips I: Changes in inpatient child psychiatry: consequences and recommendations. J Am Acad Child Adolesc Psychiatry 27:397–403, 1988

Kanner L: Child Psychiatry. Springfield, IL, Charles C Thomas, 1935

Rafferty F: Resolved: child and adolescent psychiatric practice in the twenty-first century will largely be hospital based. J Am Acad Child Adolesc Psychiatry 27:815–818, 1988

Schowalter J: Child psychiatry program directors' ratings of residency experiences. J Am Acad Child Adolesc Psychiatry 28:124–129, 1984

CHAPTER SEVENTEEN

Geriatric Psychiatry

Marion Z. Goldstein, M.D.
Kye Kim, M.D.

Meeting the Challenge

The field of aging has attracted considerable interest in the last two centuries. There has been an increasing knowledge base in the medical biology, sociology, psychology, and epidemiology of aging, especially during the past two decades, in response to the increasing numbers of elderly individuals in our population. However, geriatric psychiatry as a specialty area of clinical practice, teaching, and research is in different developmental stages in different geographic locations and institutional settings. The first training program in geriatric psychiatry was established in 1965 at Duke University; yet, in many other settings, geriatric specialty medical mental health services have as yet to be developed, and in others, these services have yet to be integrated with training or research.

Description of Geriatric Psychiatry

By definition, *geriatric psychiatry* deals with the evaluation, assessment, diagnosis, and treatment of mental disorders and disturbances in older adults and their support network. Geriatric psychiatrists have taken a leadership role in redefining the parameters of psychiatry as a medical specialty as it applies to the older adult. Geriatric psychiatrists have become valued leaders of multidisciplinary teams of nurses, psychologists, social workers, pharmacologists, occupational therapists, physician assistants, and others.

The number of psychiatrists with specialty interests, training, and knowledge in the field of aging and psychopathology of late life is increasing gradually but has not kept up with the ever-increasing demand for their participation. There is currently a great shortage of psychiatrists who have been comprehensively trained in geriatric psychiatry in medical school and residency and an even greater shortage of geriatric psychiatrists with fellowship training or equivalent experiences. In Canada, residency training programs in psychiatry are mandated to offer 3-month full-time or 6-month half-time rotations through geriatric psychiatry. This is not as yet the case in the United States. Estimates of needed geriatric psychiatrists in practice have varied, with 1,130 geriatric psychiatrists (full-time equivalent [FTE]) for 1977 and 6,155 (FTE) for 1981 quoted (Kane et al. 1980; Lazarus and Weinberg 1981).

The so-called graying of the population is a major challenge to the medical profession in general and to psychiatrists and geriatric psychiatrists in particular. The total number of elderly individuals is rising and so are the numbers requiring attention from the mental health sector to enhance quality of life during senescence. In the year 2000, it is estimated that one out of every five individuals in the United States will be age 65 and above, with those age 85 and over the fastest growing segment. The hospital population consists of more and more patients age 65 and older, and 20% of individuals age 80 and over reside in long-term care facilities (Borson et al. 1989).

Problems With Delivery of Care to Elderly Individuals

Estimates of the number of elderly individuals who have mental health problems vary widely depending on whether they live in the community; attend medical or family practice clinics; are in general hospitals or in psychiatry units in general hospitals or in private, federal, state, or county hospitals; or reside in long-term care facilities. There is a high prevalence of dementia, depression, anxiety, paranoia, and delirium among elderly individuals on medical and surgical units. These conditions remain frequently unrecognized and untreated or are relegated to an ill-perceived and outdated concept of the aging process. Estimates of the occurrence of mental illness in residents of long-term care facilities are as high as 94% (Rovner et al. 1986) and 80% or above in other studies (e.g., Borson et al. 1989). A recent community survey in Boston (Evans et al. 1989) revealed that 10% of individuals age 65 and over and 47% of individuals age 80 and over have some form of cognitive impairment. The condition of dementia is as yet not routinely and appropriately attended to by the majority of practicing physicians.

In contrast to these statistics, elderly individuals receive only 7% of all psychiatry inpatient services, 6% of community mental health services, and 2%–9% of private practice services (American Psychiatric Association 1988–1989). But, in contrast to these findings, older adults receive as much as 50% of all benzodiazepines and sedatives prescribed. Moreover, studies have shown that the frequent prescribing of psychotropic medications for elderly individuals is often inappropriate and poorly monitored by physicians who have not had the benefit of specialty training in either gerontology or geriatric psychiatry. The reality is that elderly individuals and their families are used to going to their internists, family practitioners, or other primary care physicians with physical complaints, regardless of their etiology. Many of these physical complaints mask underlying symptoms and syndromes of treatable psychiatric disorders that, according to an abundance of research findings (Barsa et al. 1986; Erkinjunitti et al. 1986; Larson et al. 1987; Patterson 1986), are overlooked, misdiagnosed and mistreated, or not followed up appropriately.

Another problem that is known to be prevalent in primary care practice is the frequent oversight of the need for medical and mental health attention by the caregivers for frail, elderly individuals. This oversight occurs despite the findings that family caregivers of the disabled elderly seek out health and mental health care in considerably higher numbers than in the noncaregiving community population. Studies have shown that as many as 50% of family caregivers of elderly individuals have manifestations of mental health disorders (Gallagher et al. 1989; Haley et al. 1987; Pruchno and Potashnik 1989).

Ageism prevails in many sectors of our society and is an attitude that geriatric psychiatrists need to detect, understand, and learn to deal with effectively in many situations. For example, from the inception of Medicare in the 1960s until 1988, Medicare reimbursement for outpatient medical mental health services received by elderly patients (i.e., patients age 65 and over) was limited to $250 per year, with the patient paying 50% of the fee out of pocket (in contrast to the 20% copayment they made for other medical services). Inpatient coverage required patients to make a 1-day copayment. After 1988, the yearly limit for Medicare reimbursement for outpatient medical mental health care was $1,100; in 1990, the upper limit was completely abolished. This financial disincentive for both patient and provider had many consequences: it contributed to 1) a lengthy delay in providing elderly individuals with the help needed to overcome the stigma they, even more than the younger population, experienced when requiring psychiatric help; 2) overuse of primary care office visits and diagnostic procedures; 3) an inability of psychiatrists in private practice to service elderly individuals appropriately before and after hospitalizations; and 4) a disincentive for psychiatrists to improve their skills and knowledge base in treating this population. Until the inception of *Current Procedural Terminology* (CPT; American Medical Association 1992) codes for evaluation and management (E/M) services, Medicare did not have a reimbursement code for contacts with families of elderly individuals, be it to obtain collateral information, assess caregiver burden, or educate to ensure compliance with recommendations made to a forgetful, depressed, or anxious elderly patient.

In 1992, Medicare instituted new *evaluation and management codes,* codes based on the nature and level of the service rendered and the length of time required to provide the service for all physicians, regardless of their specialty. The fee schedules for these services will be the product of nationally established relative value units, the geographic practice cost indices for the locale in which a service is rendered, and a national conversion factor, which is a single national number to be used by all insurance carriers in calculating payments under Medicare fee schedules. It is expected that there will be a 5-year phase-in period for this new system and that other insurance companies will eventually follow this fee schedule. A code for outpatient psychotherapy remains in the new schedule, and Medicare will continue to reimburse for this service at a 50% rate, as this is the code for nursing home psychiatric visits. Individuals as well as organized psychiatry are actively working with legislators to rectify this inequity.

Elderly individuals can, of course, have insurance that supplements Medicare reimbursement, called Medigap. As yet, these insurance carriers have to be mandated to cover the 50% copayment. These mandates can be established as the result of forceful and effective advocacy by individuals and organizations such as the American Psychiatric Association (APA).

Dealing with the bureaucracy is frustrating for those who feel disenfranchised by it—elderly individuals, their families, and providers of care—and is even a challenge to those who have been able to affect the system in a positive way.

Addressing the Challenge in Academia

Are medical school curricula, residency training programs, fellowship programs in geriatric psychiatry, and continuing medical education programs rising to the challenge of preparing a sufficient number of physicians to be caring and effective providers of the ever-increasing elderly population (Group for the Advancement of Psychiatry 1983; Marin et al. 1988)? So far, training programs in geriatric psychiatry have not kept pace with the need for specialists in geriatric psychiatry (Busse and Blazer 1989; Gaitz 1982; Kane et al. 1980; Langsley and Yager 1988; Lazarus and Weinberg 1981; Small et al. 1988; Varner and Verwoerdt 1975).

Well-trained geriatric psychiatrists are needed to establish and maintain high-quality centers for providing mental health services for elderly patients and in which medical students, psychiatry residents, residents in other medical disciplines (e.g., family practice), and fellows can learn to diagnose and treat older patients and their families. The geriatric psychiatrists in such centers have opportunities to become leaders in their field and to make major contributions to training and research efforts.

In 1980, Kane et al. estimated that by 1990 between 900 and 1,600 geriatricians and 400 geriatric psychiatrists would be needed to staff the 127 medical schools in the United States. A minimum of two full-time faculty members dedicated to geriatric psychiatry was considered to be necessary to get a geriatric psychiatry program under way. A 1984 report by the National Institute on Aging on education and training in geriatrics and gerontology suggested that by 1990 at least 600 geriatric psychiatry faculty would be required in medical schools, and that by the year 2000 that requirement would more than double to 1,300. Based on responses to a 1989 mail survey we sent to departments of psychiatry, we defined a trend among these departments toward planned increases in faculty positions for directors of divisions of geriatric psychiatry, chiefs of inpatient and outpatient geriatric psychiatry programs, and directors of training and research in geriatric psychiatry during the next 5 years. This same survey showed that rotations of medical students and residents through geriatric specialty services was as yet sporadic and not necessarily coordinated with didactic programs.

Departments of psychiatry vary widely in their initiation, programs, and commitment to service, teaching, and research in geriatric psychiatry and in their collaborations with geriatrics. The psychiatry departments with established programs of excellence not only are growing and expanding, but are also developing leaders for other programs and services. Opportunities remain abundant and varied.

In 1978, National Institute of Mental Health (NIMH) funds became available for geriatric psychiatry fellowship programs. These fellowships varied in duration from 1 to 3 years as well as in emphasis and orientation, depending on programs and mentors available. (There has been a hiatus of available funds toward these fellowships since 1988.) In addition, some states fund fellowship programs and some departments have private endowment funds. Funding for six to eight 2-year Veterans Administration geriatric psychiatry fellowships have also been made available. Some departments of psychiatry are willing to fund geriatric psychiatry fellowships out of graduate medical education funds in order to increase the number of these much needed geriatric psychiatrists as academicians and practitioners. The number of available fellowship programs has increased from 11 in 1980 to 55 in 1992.

A considerable milestone toward solidifying geriatric psychiatry as a specialty was reached by the establishment of an American Board of Psychiatry and Neurology (ABPN) Added Qualifications examination in 1991. In order to take this examination in 1991–1992, 1994, and

1995, psychiatrists had to be board certified in psychiatry and neurology and have 25% of their clinical practice devoted to elderly individuals. After 1996, applicants will be required to have completed their PGY-4 and 1 year of a Council for Graduate Medical Education (CGME)–accredited fellowship in geriatric psychiatry, which will constitute PGY-5.

Work Settings

For many psychiatrists in practice heretofore, their work setting has been the primary determinant of the percentage of elderly patients in their practice. For example, according to the 1982 APA Professional Activity Survey, international medical school graduates and psychiatrists in state hospitals saw the highest percentage of elderly patients. The 1988–1989 APA survey revealed similar findings. Recent data analyses comparing these two surveys showed that the percentage of psychiatrists whose practice comprised more than 20% elderly patients (with some practices serving more than 50% elderly patients) was slightly higher than that in the 1982 study (Goldstein et al. 1993).

Consultation-Liaison

Psychiatrists who spend a great deal of their time in doing consultation-liaison in general hospitals see a considerable number of medically ill elderly patients. A particularly satisfying part of this work setting is the liaison aspect, which gives geriatric psychiatrists an opportunity to educate their colleagues in the comprehensive care of elderly individuals and their families.

Forensics

A psychiatric skill that is of particular value to the legal system is assessment of competency. This is frequently requested to guide the legal system in determining when elderly individuals can no longer make specific decisions on their own behalf. Judges are called upon to make decisions on behalf of many elderly individuals about the need for guardianship, committee, or conservatorship (terminology differs from state to state, and refers to financial and/or health determinations the appointed person can make for the elderly individual). They require expert assessments by well-trained and experienced geriatric psychiatrists in determining whether a person is competent to consent to or to refuse treatment in cases that do not involve emergency medical decisions and in cases where no "living will" is available and there is no family who can advocate for the patient's wishes. Collaboration between the geriatric psychiatrist, family, elderly patient, and their lawyers can evolve into a rewarding and stimulating working relationship on behalf of the best interest of all concerned.

Nursing Homes

The lack of psychiatric services in nursing homes has recently received considerable attention because of new regulations that nursing homes must provide psychiatric services for patients with mental health problems. Many psychiatrists find themselves untrained to render these services, which require knowledge of psychopathology of late life stages as well as knowledge of the pharmacodynamics and pharmacokinetics of medications and combinations of medications elderly individuals are often prescribed.

Most psychiatrists who have been trained in geriatric psychiatry have found nursing home consultation-liaison a rewarding and challenging experience. Sophisticated nursing home administrators and nurses who have learned the value of specialty psychiatric consultation-liaison have contracted with psychiatrists for a weekly block of time and assume the responsibility of billing Medicare, thus relieving psychiatrists from a much disliked and time-consuming bureaucratic hassle. Such contractual arrangements with nursing homes enable medical directors and other physicians, as well as nurses in nursing homes, to request psychiatric consultations.

Multidisciplinary Teams

Specialty trained psychiatrists have been valued leaders of multidisciplinary teams in a variety of settings such as inpatient units, outpatient programs, day hospital programs, outreach programs, and community outreach programs. The complexity of psychiatric care of elderly individuals requires a team effort in order to assess appropriate community resources for elderly individuals and their families, and to conduct the initial and follow-up assessments with attention to all organs that may be vulnerable or affected by the aging process, by pathology, or by medications. It is this team effort and close contact with colleagues in different specialties that geriatric psychiatrists report finding most satisfying in their practice. The multidisciplinary team not only enables psychiatrists to render more comprehensive care, it also enables them to serve more elderly patients and families per unit time. Studies have shown that accessible and affordable specialty services for elderly individuals are well received and appropriately used.

It is quite important for psychiatrists who work in an institutional setting to gain some administrative training in the course of becoming a geriatric psychiatrist because attitudes, conscious or unconscious, of ageism on the part of those in authority and with fiscal responsibilities may not allow them to prioritize the so obviously needed services, training, or research.

Veterans Administration

The Veterans Administration has developed 15 geriatric research education and clinical centers (GRECCs). These GRECCs began to be developed in 1975 for the purpose of advancing scientific knowledge on aging and problems of elderly individuals, training medical and associated health students and practitioners, and improving the care of elderly veterans through the development of innovative clinical care models (Van Stone and Goldstein 1993).

Professional and Government Organizations

Pioneering efforts in geriatric psychiatry have gathered momentum in a variety of professional organizations. The APA's Council on Aging was established in 1971. The American Association for Geriatric Psychiatry (AAGP) was founded in 1978, and now has over

1,500 members. Both the APA's Council on Aging and the AAGP interface with the Gerontological Society of America, the American Geriatric Society, the American Association of Retired Persons, and several other organizations committed to aging and elderly individuals.

Coordination of research and training in aging on a federal level has had a major impact on moving the field forward. The Administration on Aging, created in 1965 within the U. S. Department of Health, Education, and Welfare, has as its mission the development and coordination of services and research initiatives for elderly individuals.

In the 1970s, the NIMH Center for Studies of Mental Health of the Aging and the National Institute on Aging were established. One focus of these agencies was to develop specialty training fellowships; faculty development programs; continuing education; in-service, demonstration, and research training; and curriculum projects. Funding has been uneven, especially for training and projects other than research. The National Institute on Aging was established in 1974 as part of the NIMH and was an indication of governmental recognition and support for basic research in the aging process, diseases, and psychological problems of elderly individuals and their caregivers.

Special Issues

There is a great deal of collegiality among geriatric psychiatrists and geriatricians and a great deal of mentoring. Incentives for psychiatry residents to be introduced to the field of geriatric psychiatry are available on a competitive basis. The AAGP offers an opportunity for PGY-2 psychiatry residents to be considered for sponsorship to attend the association's annual meetings for 2 years and participate in committees of their choice. The AAGP also has a booth at the APA's annual meetings where attendees can learn about the many functions of the AAGP and meet experts in the field, including directors of fellowship programs. Another opportunity is available to residents who have won an APA fellowship—they can choose to participate on APA's Council on Aging. These are stimulating and rewarding learning experiences during which professional growth and important networking take place. Most geriatric psychiatrists seem aware of the need to encourage young psychiatrists to acquire specialty knowledge and training and participate in the quest of not only adding years to life, but quality of life to years.

Because poverty all too frequently accompanies aging, many mentally ill elderly patients are served by the public health sector. Positions for psychiatrists in state hospitals often involve carrying a sizable patient population of elderly individuals. Many of these positions have been taken by international medical graduates. All psychiatrists with a large patient population of elderly individuals need to be made aware of and encouraged to acquire specialty training.

In a field that is as yet underserved, women and those from minority populations are generally welcomed. Minority elderly patients, as well as other elderly patients, seek familiarity from their caregivers and would benefit by having more caregivers available who are familiar with their particular culture. The opportunity to speak a native language is of particular importance for foreign-born elderly patients.

Women, daughters, and daughters-in-law are the notoriously overstressed, "sandwiched between two generations" caregivers of elderly individuals. More women professionals in this specialty would certainly create considerably more empathy with overburdened caregivers and lend support to efforts to advocate for reimbursement of professional time spent with families of elderly individuals. In addition, because the majority of elderly patients are women, more women in this specialty will bring more empathy for the plight of older women and what part their previous marital status and maternal role have played in the shaping of their presenting situation. Women physicians are more likely to recognize how female patients' needs for intimacy and companionship affect their medical and mental condition. Eventually, with sufficient research in that arena, a diagnostic category may even be established that categorizes levels of need for attachment and availability as risk factors for other conditions.

Women live longer than men, spend more of their aging years alone, and are more likely than men to be poor, abused, neglected, and exploited. Inadequate attention has been paid to these issues in the mental health care of elderly women to date. Furthermore, the unique problems of aging minority women have also been inadequately addressed.

Women in geriatric psychiatry are underrepresented. In 1990, the APA membership consisted of 23% women and the AAGP membership, 11% women. As in other fields, women need to mentor junior peers and network with each other in addition to collaborating with those male colleagues who will not only advance the careers of their male colleagues but also recognize the very special attributes women bring to this challenging and growing specialty.

Conclusion

Geriatric psychiatry is a field in which the demand for expertise and sensitivity will remain in excess of the supply for some years to come. It is a challenging field with an expanding knowledge base with many and varied opportunities.

References

American Medical Association: Physicians' Current Procedural Terminology, 4th Edition. Chicago, IL, AMA, 1992

American Psychiatric Association: Professional Activities Survey. Washington, DC, American Psychiatric Association, 1982

American Psychiatric Association: Professional Activities Survey. Washington, DC, American Psychiatric Association, 1988–1989

Barsa J, Toner J, Gurland B, et al: Ability of internists to recognize and manage depression in the elderly. International Journal of Geriatric Psychiatry 1:57–62, 1986

Borson S, Liptzin B, Nininger J, et al: Nursing homes and the mentally ill elderly: a task force report of the American Psychiatric Association. Washington, DC, American Psychiatric Association, 1989

Busse EW, Blazer DG: The future of geriatric psychiatry, in Geriatric Psychiatry. Edited by Busse EW, Blazer DG. Washington, DC, American Psychiatric Press, 1989, pp 671–695

Erkinjunitti I, Wikstrom J, Palo J, et al: Dementia among medical inpatients: evaluation of 2,000 consecutive admissions. Arch Intern Med 146:1923–1924, 1986

Evans DA, Funkenstein H, Albert M, et al: Prevalence of Alzheimer's disease in a community population of older persons. JAMA 126:2551–2556, 1989

Gaitz CM: The practice of geriatric psychiatry in psychosocial intervention with the aged. Psychiatr Clin North Am 5:215–227, 1982

Gallagher D, Rose J, Rivera P, et al: Prevalence of depression in family caregivers. J Am Geriatr Soc 29:449–455, 1989

Goldstein MZ, Colends CC, Kennedy GJ, et al: Selected models of practice in geriatric psychiatry (APA Task Force Report). Washington, DC, American Psychiatric Press, 1993, pp 39–44

Group for the Advancement of Psychiatry, Committee on Aging: Mental health and aging: approaches to curriculum development (Vol 11, Publication No. 114). New York, Group for the Advancement of Psychiatry, April 1983

Haley WE, Levine EG, Brown SL, et al: Psychological, social and health consequences of caring for a relative with senile dementia. J Am Geriatr Soc 35:405–411, 1987

Kane R, Solomon D, Beck J, et al: The future need for geriatric manpower in the United States. N Engl J Med 302:1327–1332, 1980

Langsley DG, Yager J: The definition of a psychiatrist: eight years later. Am J Psychiatry 145:469–475, 1988

Larson EB, Kukull WA, Buchner D, et al: Adverse drug reactions associated with global cognitive impairment in elderly persons. Ann Intern Med 107:169–173, 1987

Lazarus LW, Weinberg J: Training in geropsychiatry: problems and process. Am J Psychiatry 138:1366–1369, 1981

Marin RS, Foster J, Ford CV, et al: A curriculum for education in geriatric psychiatry. Am J Psychiatry 145:836–843, 1988

National Institute on Aging: Report on education and training in geriatrics and gerontology (NIA administrative document). February 1984

Patterson C: Iatrogenic disease in late life. Clin Geriatr Med 2:121–136, 1986

Pruchno RA, Potashnik SL: Caregiving spouses physical and mental health perspective. J Am Geriatr Soc 34:697–705, 1989

Rovner BW, Kafonek S, Filipp L, et al: Prevalence of mental illness in a community nursing home. Am J Psychiatry 143:1446–1449, 1986

Small GW, Fong K, Beck JC: Training in geriatric psychiatry: will the supply meet the demand? Am J Psychiatry 145:476–478, 1988

Van Stone WM, Goldstein MZ: Mental health services for older adults in the VA system. Hosp Community Psychiatry 44:828–830, 1993

Varner RV, Verwoerdt A: Training of psychogeriatricians, in Modern Perspectives in the Psychiatry of Old Age. Edited by Howell JG. New York, Brunner/Mazel, 1975, pp 570–583

CHAPTER EIGHTEEN

Forensic Psychiatry

Naomi Goldstein, M.D.
Thomas G. Gutheil, M.D.

Front-page headlines blaring "Battle of the Experts" conjure up images of affluent hired guns, bringing shame to the noble psychiatric profession. This image problem is unfortunate. The insanity defense is one of the more visible forensic issues, but its public prominence and media-based significance are disproportionate to its modest place in the broad spectrum of forensic practice.

There are enormous needs and opportunities for knowledgeable and experienced psychiatrists willing to bring their expertise into nonmedical arenas, including civil and criminal courtrooms, prisons, hospitals, insurance companies, legislative offices, and even the chambers of judges who must determine patients' right to treatment or the adequacy of prison mental health programs.

Although noxious headlines reflect very real issues, most psychiatrists today, whether self-identified as forensic psychiatrists or not, at some time in their careers offer forensic opinions: determining a patient's dangerousness, deciding whether legal criteria for commitment or release have been met, determining competency of patients to refuse treatment, and estimating disability. Many other psychiatrists also work in prisons and jails or consult with courts and probation departments. Hence, forensic issues impinge on general psychiatry in many ways.

Definition and History

The forensic psychiatrist is one who has developed expertise in the areas of psychiatry and law, spends substantial time in the forensic arena, and is comfortable in a range of nonmedical settings. Many forensic psychiatrists also spend significant amounts of time in non-forensic settings, treatment settings, or private practice (Hanson et al. 1984; Robitscher 1978).

Forensic psychiatry emerged during the 19th century as legal thinking about the impact of psychological processes on criminal activity became increasingly sophisticated, and psychiatry, then emerging as a specialty, placed itself increasingly on a scientific basis. The notion that having a mental disorder is a reason for exoneration from guilt is an ancient one, but a psychiatric formulation of this principle awaited the thinking of the great American psychiatrist, Isaac Ray, fourth president of the American Psychiatric Association (APA). In 1843, the British courts fashioned an insanity defense known as the M'Naghten Rule, which was rapidly adopted in the United States and elsewhere. Whether modernized, expanded, or narrowed, this rule has been maintained as a central element in Western legal thinking.

In a movement toward broadening psychiatric participation in the criminal justice system in the 20th century, great psychiatric leaders such as Karl Menninger recommended that psychiatric expertise be made available in all courtrooms for evaluation of offenders concerning issues quite unrelated to guilt or innocence. Leading psychiatrists had long since begun to concern themselves with the nature of criminality, to work in prisons, and to treat offenders.

Paralleling the expansion of psychiatry itself, civil law involving psychiatric expertise was developed; this field now includes personal injury litigation; evaluation of disability for soldiers, veterans, and injured workers; and juvenile and family law. By the mid-20th century, however, the impact of critics of psychiatry such as Thomas Szasz, a forensic psychiatrist, and of the emerging civil rights movement with its interest in disenfranchised minority populations, led to a profound reexamination of involuntary commitment, the right to treatment or to refuse treatment, informed consent, access to records, and other civil liberties for psychiatric patients. Psychiatrists were forced to focus more acutely on the legal, ethical, and moral as well as clinical bases for much of what they did. It is forensic psychiatrists who study these broader issues, teaching, writing, and advocating in the public arena as well as to the profession.

Thus, the scope of forensic psychiatry eventually broadened from being the application of psychiatry to legal issues for legal ends to embracing a whole range of issues covered by the term *psychiatry and the law*. In 1988, the American Board of Forensic Psychiatry, founded in 1976 to grant subspecialty certification, defined forensic psychiatry as "a subspecialty in which scientific and clinical expertise is applied to legal issues in legal contexts embracing civil, criminal, correctional or legislative matters, which should be practiced in accordance with guidelines and ethical principles enunciated by the profession of psychiatry."

Forensic Psychiatry Organizations

The discipline of forensic psychiatry has been strongly supported by organized psychiatry. In 1924, William Alanson White established a small but prestigious committee within the APA to study relationships between psychiatry and the law. In 1951, the APA offered the first of its two major awards for a substantial contribution to understanding the interface between psychiatry and the law. In 1969, the American Academy of Psychiatry and the Law (AAPL) was organized to further forensic education and the quality of practice. AAPL now has about 1,400 members, including both forensic practitioners and psychiatrists interested in forensic issues. During the 1970s, the APA established two major organizational components in addition to other committees to address issues around psychiatry and the law. And, in 1990, the APA once more had a president, Elissa P. Benedek, who, like Isaac Ray in 1844, was clearly identified as a forensic psychiatrist.

Other organizations devoted solely to forensic issues have appeared, and a vast literature, including numerous forensic journals and bulletins, as well as distinguished awards in the field have emerged. The purpose of these organizations has been to encourage education and ethical practice and to improve the level of competency in forensic matters, particularly for psychiatrists wishing to specialize.

In 1991, the APA endorsed forensic psychiatry as a subspecialty, subject to an examination for "added qualifications" by the American Board of Neurology and Psychiatry; the first such examination occurred in October 1994. In defining forensic psychiatry, the APA identified three areas of competence and knowledge: 1) the use of psychiatric information in resolving legal matters, 2) the legal regulation of psychiatric practice, and 3) the treatment of patients in special settings—that is, jails, prisons, and maximum security institutions.

Criteria for and Training as a Forensic Psychiatrist

Historically, the basic requirement for forensic work is to be a good clinician. Many lawyers have assiduously avoided retaining experts who are known only as forensic experts and who might be perceived as "tainted" or "hired guns." Yet both lawyers and courts have recognized the need for the services of clinically experienced, credible experts who understand the need for a forensic opinion, who are familiar with and willing to work with the legal criteria and to offer opinions in nonmedical settings. Most ethical lawyers ask psychiatrists for an independent opinion and then live and work with that opinion. Most forensic work remains behind the scenes, is used in civil and criminal negotiations, and may also be used to provide or obtain appropriate help or treatment for an individual.

For those readers considering specialization in forensic psychiatry, a variety of training opportunities exist. As of 1994, there were 32 forensic fellowships in the United States and Canada, with other programs under development (Pollack 1985). Sixteen of these fellowships have been accredited by AAPL's Accreditation Council on Fellowships in Forensic Psychiatry, which is cosponsored by the American Academy of Forensic Sciences (AAPL 1994). These accredited fellowships, as well as some of the others, are full-time, 1-year programs. They provide a range of training experiences in domestic relations, civil and criminal matters, and outpatient, inpatient, and correctional settings. Training includes hands-on experience in evaluation, report writing, and testifying, as well as didactic and practical attention to the regulation of psychiatry and to ethical and historical issues (Pollack 1985). In considering a particular program, a potential forensic psychiatrist should determine whether it is a broad-based program and should maintain an open mind about career options, as there are many. Eventually, a fellowship in forensic psychiatry will be a prerequisite for examination for "added qualifications" given by the American Board of Psychiatry and Neurology. As of 1993, it was not clear which training programs would ultimately be approved and which accrediting body would approve them.

The "Stuff" of Forensic Psychiatry

Forensic psychiatry offers a range of career opportunities for men and women equally, with positions available on a part-time or full-time basis, reimbursed by private or public funds, and located within the private or public sector. A forensic psychiatrist may provide clinical evaluation and treatment, consult, teach, write, administer, or testify. Although some forensic experts are also lawyers, and although all forensic psychiatrists should be familiar with relevant law, forensic psychiatrists are called upon for broad knowledge and skills in psychiatry, not to cite case law, make rulings or decisions, or decide actual case outcomes. Good forensic psychiatrists bring together the best in psychiatry in the service of the functioning of the law (Appelbaum and Gutheil 1991; Simon 1989).

The demands of forensic practice have expanded considerably, and psychiatrists are frequently involved in several different areas of practice. Except where the psychiatrist remains clearly in a treatment relationship, the forensic psychiatrist's role is essentially consultative (Bloom and Bloom 1985).

Forensic psychiatry practice may be broken down into various areas of interest.

Civil Law

Personal injury or tort litigation. In personal injury (often called *psychic injury* or *trauma*) suits, psychiatric experts may evaluate claims for mental damages. Posttraumatic stress disorder, now recognized as a distinct diagnostic entity, or other psychiatric diagnoses, such as major depression, are the common subjects of such litigation.

Malpractice and related claims. Expertise may be needed to evaluate psychic trauma in cases of malpractice by other physicians, including psychiatrists. In psychiatric practice, failure to obtain informed consent, commitment without proper indications, breach of confidentiality, and sexual misconduct with a patient involve a group of issues called *intentional torts*. In evaluating malpractice, the psychiatrist is guided by "the four Ds": a *Duty* must have been established between physician and patient; there must have been a *Dereliction* of this duty; there must be *Damages;* and the damages must be *Directly* caused by the dereliction of duty (Gutheil 1989).

> A patient is sexually molested by a physician in the course of a medical contact. Was there a doctor-patient relationship? Was this a breach of the doctor-patient relationship? What were the psychiatric damages if any; that is, is there any diagnosable psychiatric disorder, is the former patient impaired, and was this due to the sexual abuse?

Disability and workers' compensation. Psychiatrists are needed to evaluate mental disability for many purposes; occasionally they perform these evaluations in their routine practice. Because many treating psychiatrists justly fear that involvement in advocacy might interfere with treatment, independent experts are routinely retained to make some of these evaluations, either as consultants or as regular agency employees.

Competency. Although *competency* used to be a term referring to global functioning, today it is specific to a particular decision. Psychiatrists may be asked to evaluate a person for competency to handle funds, to make a will, to get married, to make a contract, or to give informed consent or refusal of treatment. Evaluations are also used in criminal situations (see the section on criminal law below). In most instances, the criteria for competency flow logically from the issue itself, though competency may also be defined more precisely by courts.

> A depressed, handicapped woman on a respirator for life support asked to have the respirator shut off. Does she understand her options and the outcomes? Is this to be considered a suicide?

> A family is dismayed to discover that a man with a history of manic-depressive illness has been buying extraordinary businesses with large sums of family money. Did his bipolar illness so interfere with his judgment that the contracts should be nullified?

In such situations, psychiatrists evaluate and render opinions about mental diseases or defects, or degrees of impairment affecting cognition, judgment, and reality testing with regard to specific criteria defined by statute or case law. Although forensic psychiatrists must be familiar with these criteria in rendering opinions, ultimate decisions are made by judge or jury.

Miscellaneous. Psychiatrists have long been asked to make difficult decisions, some with major political or moral connotations. For example, will a mother's life be endangered if she carries a pregnancy to term? What is the impact of abortion or of carrying an unwanted pregnancy? What is the impact of sexual harassment or discrimination in the workplace? Should an individual be excused from military service for psychiatric disorders? Recently, forensic psychiatrists have been called to evaluate the emotional impact of environmental or occupational hazards and to assess the impact of major disasters. Psychiatric input can be critical in guiding the court in such cases.

Divorce and Custody Cases

Psychiatrists and psychologists are frequently involved in the evaluation of families and children to determine which party should be awarded custody of the children. The theory of custody itself changes over time to reflect evolving mores. Most recently, guidelines have focused on determining what is "in the best interest of the child," with the father occasionally becoming the custodial parent or with joint custody arrangements being designed.

Psychiatrists may also be asked to evaluate a parent's competency to be a parent, as when a mentally ill mother says she cannot cope with the children, or when a mother with a poor clinical history wishes to retrieve children from a good foster home or from adoptive parents.

Spousal and child abuse and incest generate very difficult evaluations in the family court setting, where custody decisions depend on the establishment of such patterns. Spouses seeking custody may exaggerate or fabricate allegations of sexual abuse, posing a diagnostic challenge.

Criminal Law

Although occasional headlines on notorious criminal cases that involved psychiatric testimony may cause much resentment among the profession and the citizenry, thousands of useful psychiatric evaluations in the criminal court setting are done yearly with no publicity.

Competency to stand trial. Psychiatrists evaluate defendants for competency to be arraigned, plead, go to trial, or be sentenced. Criteria for competency are generally codified in law under criminal procedure. The psychiatrist is asked whether the individual, as a result of a mental disease or defect, lacks the capacity to understand the charges and proceedings against him or her and/or to cooperate in his or her own defense, as in the following example:

> A 45-year-old mentally ill man assaults a security guard at a hospital. The lawyer cannot work with this client and requests "consultation" through determination of trial competency. The psychiatrist determines that the client has a long-standing schizoaffective disorder in acute exacerbation. He is too agitated, preoccupied, hostile, paranoid, and out of contact with reality to cooperate with his lawyer in his defense, although he clearly understands the nature of the charges and proceedings. The psychiatrist advises the court that, in her opinion, the defendant is not competent and that psychiatric hospitalization is indicated for treatment and restoration to competency.

In cases involving minor crimes, the court may be amenable to psychiatric disposition of a case and has the option of deferring prosecution with the understanding that the individual must be treated. Such diversion is usually not available in the face of serious crimes, but even within the prison system psychiatrists can advocate for and provide psychiatric care.

Criminal responsibility. The *Hinckley* case, in which the defendant was accused of shooting then President Ronald Reagan and was declared not guilty by reason of insanity, was seen by some as a disaster for psychiatry's image; it led to attempts to tighten insanity defense statutes nationwide. The *insanity defense,* a profound moral notion within the law, has been expressed in a variety of statutory wordings, but in general it represents exoneration from responsibility if the person, as a result of mental disease or defect, lacks the capacity to understand the nature, wrongfulness, and consequences of the alleged crime. Each jurisdiction has its own set of insanity defense criteria or statutes. Use of a psychiatrist to make the requisite diagnoses illustrates the common-law principle that experts be permitted to testify if such testimony will enhance a jury's knowledge of an issue about which a layperson is not knowledgeable. As with incompetency, the ultimate decision rests with the judge or jury.

> A 23-year-old male with no criminal record and several psychiatric hospitalizations struck a prostitute on the head with a hammer and killed her, then had sex with her, and cooked parts of her body before being arrested. He told police that a voice had told him that the prostitute was the devil and was poisoning him. The psychiatrist was asked to give an opinion about whether this individual had a mental disease or defect and to determine if this individual, as a result of mental disease or defect, lacked the capacity to appreciate the nature, consequences, and/or wrongfulness of what he was doing.

Successful insanity defenses are relatively infrequent; acquittal on this basis usually leads to hospitalization and reevaluation to determine potential dangerousness and further psychiatric needs.

Sentencing and other evaluations. Psychiatrists also evaluate defendants for their general mental state and for sentencing purposes. Many criminal courts have created on-site psychiatric clinics or specifically retain psychiatrists to perform these evaluations on a regular basis. The psychiatrist's function is to give the court some idea of relevant psychiatric or mental health problems that might impact on sentencing and to make recommendations for treatment, if appropriate.

The death penalty. There are two issues with respect to the death penalty that involve psychiatric expertise.

- **Competency**—Although logic quails before the question of what it means to be competent to be executed, psychiatrists have been asked this question by the courts. Psychiatrists who must evaluate for competency and treat psychosis or depression to restore a person to competency so that execution can proceed face a nightmarish (but fortunately quite rare) ethical and moral dilemma (Bonnie 1984). Participation by the psychiatrist may be framed by both personal belief and policy determined by the medical profession.

- **Mitigation**—More satisfying for the psychiatrist is investigation into mitigating circumstances, which, by law in many states, preclude application of the death penalty and instead provide for appropriate prison sentence and possible treatment. Such circumstances might be a history of physical abuse, lack of treatment at appropriate times, or a history of mental illness or retardation.

Juvenile criminal cases. Traditionally, youths have been handled in legal contexts that downplay the adversarial dimension of the law in favor of social and psychological evaluation and informal management. Court clinics use the services of psychiatrists and other mental health professionals. Psychiatrists evaluate juvenile defendants for competency, responsibility, and disposition. Although the psychiatrist's role is the same as in evaluating adult defendants, additional troublesome questions arise: At what age is a child competent to stand trial? Is a 10-year-old bank robber to be held responsible? How about an 8-year-old who kills his little sister with a gun? When is a juvenile defendant to be treated as an adult?

Commitment, the Right to Treatment, and the Right to Refuse Treatment

Most hospital psychiatrists take commitment law and proceedings for granted, as long as the decision to commit, and often to release, is decided by a judge. At the heart of this procedure lies a forensic conclusory issue; that is, the psychiatrist must apply a medical opinion to a civil statute, an opinion often involving a prediction of dangerousness.

Numerous court decisions, including several major U.S. Supreme Court cases, have addressed the issues of the "right to treatment" and "right to refuse treatment," questions impacting broadly on psychiatric practice. The chance to study such issues, to participate in the development of briefs on these topics with lawyers and the judiciary, and to teach about practical and ethical matters have made for extremely stimulating career opportunities for psychiatrists. Malpractice implications in these concepts are substantial. Renewed recognition of all the rights of patients, particularly those of inpatients, has brought with it not only conflict and stress for psychiatrists, but a new and potentially more positive relationship with patients.

Consultation and Treatment of Offenders: Working With Probation and Parole and in the Correctional Setting

Psychiatrists consult with, and are often employed by, probation and parole departments through court clinics. Their role is to evaluate and sometimes treat individuals in clinics, the community, substance abuse programs, and forensic hospitals. This type of work provides a substantial opportunity to prevent further criminal behavior by resolving relevant psychiatric issues.

Although jails and prisons have always had their share of psychiatrically ill inmates, their numbers have swollen in this era of deinstitutionalization and homelessness. These inmates present with a broad spectrum of psychiatric diagnoses and serious substance abuse. Psychiatrists are desperately needed within these institutions to develop mental health programs, advocate for proper care for mentally ill prisoners, provide treatment, and aid in release planning and assessment of dangerousness. Special mental health programs have been designed for offenders with mental disorders and have become important components of rehabilitation programs of better institutions.

> A two-time rapist is up for parole. He has worked well in a special treatment program and has been a model prisoner. The parole board needs help in assessing dangerousness. Is he safe? How can treatment success be measured?

Misunderstanding and mismanagement of mentally ill, emotionally disturbed, and mentally retarded offenders are tragically commonplace. The dual responsibility of psychiatrists to patients and to the public is nowhere felt more keenly than in prisons; yet, even in this "foreign" setting, where security for all is the number one priority, practitioners can care for people within an ethical framework. The responsibilities of prison psychiatrists vary considerably, but range from evaluation for a wide range of purposes to treatment planning and even psychoanalytic psychotherapy. Work in the correctional setting can be stressful but is often very rewarding, offering an opportunity for almost every type of competent psychiatric practice.

Terrorism, Hostage Situations, Victimization, and Violence

Some forensic psychiatrists have experience with terrorism and perform services for government agencies in this country and abroad. A natural outgrowth of forensic work with hostage situations is the handling of an individual hostage or working with police in such crises. Often, psychiatrists have studied victimization and family and sexual violence. Although the handling of violent individuals is hardly the province of forensic psychiatrists alone, they are relied on regularly to understand and predict dangerousness as well as to handle it.

Psychiatry and the Law

The psychiatrist's ordinary clinical practice is influenced and affected by regulation and law to a surprising extent. This impact may include issues such as the number of mental health visits provided in a health maintenance organization, the extent of coverage under an indemnity plan, the right of a patient to access records, informed consent, clarification of boundary issues, or the obligation of the psychiatrist to warn potential victims of violence. Psychiatrists participate in the development of mental health codes and frequently are involved in drafting the mental health portions of class action suits applied to correctional and hospital facilities. Psychiatrists become part of inspection teams for correctional facilities to monitor compliance with these class actions. Forensic psychiatrists, in the public and private sector, have worked with state regulatory agencies and statutory bodies to develop the range of provisions that impact on patient care and psychiatric practice. This work offers a significant opportunity to teach, draft, and advocate.

Research

Forensic psychiatry offers research opportunities in areas essential for addressing broad moral and social questions, such as the impact of the insanity defense, prediction of dangerousness, understanding of malingering, or the validity of posttraumatic stress disorder as a diagnosis. Funds are available and positions have been offered in various training programs, fellowships, and other settings for such research.

The Challenges

Forensic psychiatrists have been sharply criticized for exposing to the public and media the alleged "defects" in psychiatric thinking—its subjectivity, its lack of hard science, and its ambiguities—and for promoting themselves and their pocketbooks. Unpleasant as the subject is, forensic work raises serious, unavoidable questions as to the credibility and validity of psychiatry. Even as psychiatrists develop more consistent observation techniques and diagnostic formulations, increase their knowledge about the scientific etiology of mental disorders, and develop a more sophisticated treatment armamentarium, psychiatry remains a clinical art in which the objects of inquiry are highly variable and dynamic in presentation. Experience, however, confirms that psychiatric clinicians can assess individuals and issues a layperson cannot and can offer valuable and useful opinions to the "lay world" with some consistency.

All final decisions in psychiatry are influenced by subjective data; one's personal beliefs and attitudes may clearly influence conclusions. Forensic psychiatrists, in particular, struggle with conclusions that are felt to be moral ones, properly belonging to juries. These struggles are shared by courts, philosophers, and theoreticians, but forensic psychiatrists themselves struggle hardest when they attempt to apply psychiatric findings to alien legal criteria that will ultimately be used to make social and moral judgments.

An additional challenge stems from the fact that the environment in which forensic experts work may be experienced negatively. This environment may be nonmedical, as in insurance companies, court clinics, or prisons. Even worse, forensic experts in court will be confronted by adversarial lawyers and judges whose job it is to challenge, cross-examine, and break down psychiatrists' conclusions, clinical judgment, and/or credibility. This experience can be very unpleasant if taken personally. If psychiatrists have done careful evaluations and preparation with a lawyer, have learned what to expect, and advocate only for their findings and opinions rather than for the ultimate outcome, their role is not only easier but actively rewarding. Psychiatrists who are truly committed to forensic work do not lose their medical identity, even in courtrooms.

Forensic work has many challenges. The most important qualification in forensic work is to have excellent clinical skills: for interviewing; for evaluating; for making diagnoses and forensic formulations; for planning treatments; and for applying psychodynamic theory to the understanding of symptom formation, resistance, and motivation. A wealth of interesting clinical material may be seen: not typical psychiatric patients or issues, but subjects who challenge the diagnostic manual and teach respect both for the difficulties inherent in psychiatry and for the startling variability of human behavior. Equally challenging are lawyers' questions on issues psychiatrists take for granted, questions that may lead to profound debate as to where mental illness stops and normalcy begins. The range of intellectual, ethical, and professional challenges in forensic work is breathtaking—challenges to make us think more sharply about our professional beliefs and behavior (Dietz 1987).

Forensic psychiatrists working within prisons may have substantial impact on the "mental health" of the prison itself, on policy, and in reduction of violence as well as in provision of mental health services. There are ample opportunities for research.

Lastly, forensic psychiatry offers a magnificent opportunity for teaching, generally to a receptive, interested audience—whether this consist of a judge, jury, lawyer, prison warden, or other professionals. Forensic consultation with integrity in the nonmedical world provides a superb opportunity to apply psychiatric expertise.

References

American Academy of Psychiatry and the Law, Association of Directors of Forensic Psychiatry Fellowships: Directory of Forensic Psychiatry Fellowships. Bloomfield, CT, AAPL, 1994

Appelbaum PS, Gutheil TG: The Clinical Handbook of Psychiatry and the Law, 2nd Edition. Baltimore, MD, Williams & Wilkins, 1991

Bloom JD, Bloom JL: The consultation model and forensic psychiatric practice. Bull Am Acad Psychiatry Law 13:159–164, 1985

Bonnie RJ: Morality, equality and expertise: renegotiating the relationship between psychiatry and the criminal law. Bull Am Acad Psychiatry Law 12:5–20, 1984

Dietz PE: The forensic psychiatrist of the future. Bull Am Acad Psychiatry Law 15:217–227, 1987

Gutheil TG: Legal issues in psychiatry, in Comprehensive Textbook of Psychiatry/V, 5th Edition, Vol 2. Edited by Kaplan HI, Sadock BJ. Baltimore, MD, Williams & Wilkins, 1989, pp 2107–2124

Hanson CD, Sadoff RL, Sager P, et al: Comprehensive survey of forensic psychiatrists: their training and practice. Bull Am Acad Psychiatry Law 12:403–410, 1984

Pollack S: Observations on the outcome of specialty education and training in forensic psychiatry. Bull Am Acad Psychiatry Law 13:113–119, 1985

Robitscher J: The many faces of forensic psychiatry. Bull Am Acad Psychiatry Law 6:209–213, 1978

Simon RI (ed): Annual Review of Clinical Psychiatry and the Law. Washington, DC, American Psychiatric Press, 1989

CHAPTER NINETEEN

Addiction Psychiatry

Sheila B. Blume, M.D.

Introduction

Alcoholism is the single most common mental disorder in the adult population of the United States today. This important finding of the Epidemiologic Catchment Area (ECA) survey (Regier et al. 1984) is true both for lifetime prevalence (Robins et al. 1984) and for 6-month prevalence (Meyers et al. 1984). The lifetime prevalence for alcohol abuse or dependence for American adults was found to be 13.5% and the 6-month prevalence, 4.8%. For other abuse or dependence on other drugs, the lifetime prevalence was 6.1% and the 6-month prevalence, 1.2% (Regier et al. 1990). Moreover, those who abuse alcohol and drugs often have more than one psychiatric disorder.[1]

Recent research has shown that adults who abuse alcohol are significantly more likely to have a second psychiatric disorder (i.e., *dual diagnosis*) than are individuals with non–substance-related disorders. Helzer and Pryzbeck (1988), using data from all five sites of the ECA survey, including more than 20,000 adults, found that among individuals with a lifetime diagnosis of alcohol abuse or dependence, 47% had another psychiatric diagnosis. Nearly all diagnoses were overrepresented in this group, but the most frequent were drug abuse or dependence, phobic disorder, major depression, antisocial personality, mania, and panic disorder. Helzer and Pryzbeck also found that

---

[1] Note on terminology: There are a number of terms commonly used to refer to the psychoactive substance use disorders. Recently, efforts have been made to clarify their meanings (for example, see Rinaldi et al. 1988). For the purpose of this chapter, I will use the term "chemical dependency" to include both alcohol and other drug use disorders.

alcoholic patients with additional diagnoses were more likely to have undergone treatment. These findings confirm what we as psychiatrists already know from clinical experience. Psychiatrists working in any clinical setting will be caring for patients with substance use disorders, both as a single illness and as part of a multiple disorder. Every psychiatrist should, therefore, be knowledgeable about addictions.

Furthermore, patients who are not themselves chemically dependent are often related to others who are. The Children of Alcoholics Foundation, working from national survey data, estimated that 28 million Americans, or 1 in 8 of the population, are the offspring of a parent with some alcohol problem (Russell et al. 1985). Children of alcoholic parents are well known to be at increased risk for chemical dependencies but are also at risk for a wide variety of other problems, including depression, eating disorders, attention-deficit disorder, conduct disorders in childhood, and a characteristic syndrome of intra- and interpersonal problems sometimes referred to as *codependence* (Cermak 1986). Successful psychiatric treatment of any of these disorders will be greatly enhanced by a knowledge of the family dynamics associated with alcoholism. For this reason as well, every psychiatrist should be well trained in the diagnosis and treatment of chemical dependencies.

In this chapter, however, I look beyond the general proficiency required of every practicing psychiatrist to consideration of choosing to specialize in treating chemical dependency as a career. What kind of work settings might be encountered? What roles do psychiatrists play in chemical dependency treatment vis-à-vis other physicians and health professionals? What opportunities are there for training? For teaching? For research? What are the personal rewards and sacrifices involved?

I will do my best to address these questions from the personal perspective of a psychiatrist who began to take a special interest in alcoholism during the first week of my residency training and who has worked in the field since 1962 (Blume 1986a). I have worked in the public and private sectors, in government, and, for a brief time, as medical director of the National Council on Alcoholism.

During the period 1962 to the present, there have been profound changes in both public and professional understanding and response to alcohol and drug problems. In the 1980s, a growing movement toward medical subspecialization culminated in the establishment of added qualifications in addiction psychiatry by the American Board of Psychiatry and Neurology (ABPN). The first examination for this certification, given in 1993, was taken by more than 600 psychiatrists. Other medical specialties, including internal medicine, family medicine, and preventive medicine, are also considering subspecialization. The American Society of Addiction Medicine (ASAM) has had a national certification examination since 1986. As of 1993, more than 2,600 physicians had passed this examination. Typical of periods of growth and change, there is both uncertainty and opportunity in the addiction field at present.

Historical Considerations

Psychiatrists have played a leading role in the development of addiction medicine. The disease concept of alcoholism, an idea with its roots in the ancient world, was developed and articulated by Dr. Benjamin Rush, the father of American psychiatry, in the late 18th century (Jellinek 1960). However, the turmoil surrounding the enactment and repeal of prohibition in the late 19th and early 20th centuries submerged scientific interest in alcoholism and its treatment. It was not until the late 1930s, after the founding of Alcoholics Anonymous brought renewed hope of recovery to alcoholic members, that medical attention again focused on alcoholism as a treatable disease rather than as a symptom of some other illness, a moral weakness, or a hopeless death warrant. The National Council on Alcoholism and Drug Dependence, the primary voluntary health organization concerned with alcohol and drug problems, was founded in 1944. Its first medical director, Dr. Ruth Fox, was a psychiatrist. Dr. Fox was to a great extent responsible for introducing the drug disulfiram (Antabuse) for treating alcoholism in this country. She also introduced psychodrama into alcoholism treatment.

Dr. Fox was the founding president of the New York Medical Society on Alcoholism, which was established in 1954, later renamed the American Medical Society on Alcoholism and Other Drug Dependencies, and in 1989 renamed again as the American Society of

Addiction Medicine (ASAM). Since 1988, ASAM has had a seat in the American Medical Association's (AMA's) House of Delegates as a specialty society. Psychiatrists make up approximately one-third of ASAM's membership and have been well represented among the society's leaders.

The Chemical Dependency Treatment System

Comprehensive treatment of chemical dependency involves both inpatient and outpatient care. General hospital and psychiatric hospital units and some freestanding inpatient facilities carry out detoxification and acute care for substance-induced psychoses, pathological intoxication, and other related disorders (Blume 1982). Inpatient rehabilitation programs are located in a similar variety of settings. Some specialize in the care of the dual diagnosis patient or in the treatment of adolescents. These inpatient units routinely employ a multidisciplinary treatment team approach.

The role of the psychiatrist in the inpatient program varies widely with the setting and unit. In some units, a psychiatrist is chief of service or medical director and is directly responsible for the treatment of each patient, functioning as leader of the treatment team. In others, an internist or a family physician is the medical director, and the psychiatrist functions more as a consultant on difficult cases and for patients who may have additional psychiatric diagnoses.

In either case, much of the everyday group and individual treatment is performed by counselors, who are credentialed in many states as alcoholism, addiction, or chemical dependency counselors. These counselors are well trained in working with chemically dependent people, but most do not have extensive education in abnormal psychology and psychodynamics. Many counselors are themselves recovering alcoholics or addicts or are from families affected by chemical dependency. They often have personal experience with 12-step self-help programs such as Alcoholics Anonymous, Narcotics Anonymous, Gamblers Anonymous, Al-Anon, Alateen, groups for adult children of alcoholics (ACOAs), and many others.

Working with counselors and self-help group volunteers is a challenging but rewarding experience for a psychiatrist. There are great opportunities for teaching and learning. The psychiatrist may encounter skepticism or mistrust among self-help group members who have had negative experiences with psychiatric treatment. These experiences usually involved a missed or delayed diagnosis of addiction while the psychiatrist treated the individual ineffectively for something else. Sometimes a second dependence on sedatives or benzodiazepines was iatrogenically added to the original addiction. The psychiatrist can overcome this mistrust by demonstrating a solid understanding of the addictive process and by attending meetings and learning how self-help groups work. In time, the differences between the various psychotherapeutic drugs and their potential for abuse can be communicated, to the advantage of the program's patients.

Psychiatrists specializing in chemical dependency also work more closely with primary care physicians and medical nurses than many of their colleagues. The many and varied medical complications of addictive disease invite a sustained interest in internal medicine.

Outpatient treatment varies greatly in setting and intensity. Many psychiatrists in private practice treat chemical dependency using individual, group, and family therapies. Detoxification from alcohol and certain drugs can be safely accomplished on an outpatient basis for some patients. Its feasibility depends on the severity of withdrawal and the availability of a reliable family member to provide support. Outpatient psychotherapy combined with self-help participation is a successful approach for many patients (Blume 1984; Zimberg 1982).

Outpatient clinic services vary in structure and intensity. Intensive day programs and evening and weekend programs are available in some areas. These follow a multidisciplinary team approach much like the inpatient models, and the psychiatrist's role is similar. Less frequent visits are characteristic of most outpatient clinics. However, outpatient programs often offer an educational series of lectures and discussions for patients and families and also provide space for self-help meetings on site. The psychiatrist may take part in these activities in addition to assuming a primary role in the assessment and diagnosis of new patients, treatment planning, staff supervision, and patient treatment. If disulfiram is used, the psychiatrist will often be involved in ongoing supervision of its prescription and use.

The methadone treatment clinic is a specialized facility for the outpatient care of those addicted to opiates. Because this treatment requires close medical supervision, a psychiatrist may be involved in assessing patient progress and establishing and adjusting methadone dosages, in addition to the other treatment functions mentioned above.

Because research into alcohol and drug problems is a relatively new area of inquiry, there are many important clinical questions awaiting investigation. Clinical psychiatrists with an interest in research can add to the current knowledge base in creative ways, drawing from their patient population. Federal funding for research is administered by the National Institute on Alcohol Abuse and Alcoholism (NIAAA) and the National Institute on Drug Abuse (NIDA).

Growth of the Treatment System

Recent years have brought rapid growth in the chemical dependency treatment system, along with a shift in administrative auspices. Whereas in the 1970s nearly two-thirds of existing inpatient hospital programs were operated by government bodies (e.g., Veterans Administration, state, county, township, or city agencies), this proportion had decreased to 20% by 1987 (National Institute on Alcohol Abuse and Alcoholism 1987; National Institute on Drug Abuse 1989). At the same time, the proportion of beds in investor-owned, for-profit facilities nearly tripled, from 5% in 1978 to 14.3% of the total in 1987. The proportion of beds in nongovernment, nonprofit programs increased from 31% to 66% over the same period. The growth of the nongovernment sector has been greatly encouraged by improvements in insurance coverage for chemical dependency. Collective bargaining and the education of decision makers in government and industry have accelerated this trend. Legal mandates in some states have required such coverage.

Including both inpatients and outpatients in specialized chemical dependency programs, there were approximately 812,000 Americans in treatment on October 30, 1991 (National Institute on Drug Abuse 1992). These data were derived from the National Drug and Alcoholism Treatment Unit Survey (NDATUS) of patients in treatment, which was conducted by NIAAA and NIDA at several-year intervals. The 1992 total represented a 280% increase over the 1982 total of about 290,000 patients. Of the 812,000 patients in treatment in 1992, 11% were in inpatient or residential facilities and 88% were active outpatients.

Thus, it is fair to conclude that opportunities to work in the chemical dependency treatment system will be available in the years to come. Positions in for-profit programs have increased most rapidly, but nonprofit and government-run programs are also likely to expand in the future. Private group practice will also continue to be a viable option for psychiatrists with a special interest in chemical dependency. Although the improvements in health insurance coverage mentioned above have recently been tempered by tighter restrictions and controls on length of stay, a growing public awareness of the need for these services is likely to ensure the basic integrity of the treatment system.

Professional Organizations

American Society of Addiction Medicine

The largest of the organizations for physicians treating chemical dependencies is ASAM, with more than 3,400 physician members as of 1993. Although the society's original emphasis was primarily on alcohol-related problems, the society underwent an important expansion in the early 1980s as a result of an AMA initiative that recognized the need for a medical society devoted equally to all chemical dependency problems.

One major function of the society is the sponsorship of an annual medical-scientific conference, which is preceded by the Ruth Fox Course, a popular full-day physicians' update. In addition, the society sponsors comprehensive review courses in addiction medicine at locations around the country in connection with its certification examination. ASAM has sponsored national conferences on the relationship between acquired immunodeficiency syndrome (AIDS) and chemical dependency, on tobacco dependency, and on other subjects of current importance.

ASAM is a lively organization at which problems affecting treatment are studied in depth in many committees. The society publishes the *Journal of Addictive Diseases* and has produced publications on the treatment of AIDS in chemical dependency programs and on confidentiality of alcohol and drug patient records, among other topics. The society is also active in the national policy arena.

ASAM's certification process began with an initiative from the California Society for the Treatment of Alcoholism and Other Drug Dependency, which sponsored two comprehensive examinations for California. Working from this base, ASAM developed a national examination, first given in 1986. The history and content of the examination have been described by Galanter (1985) and Bean-Bayog et al. (1985). Along with developing the examination and review course, ASAM has vigorously encouraged the establishment of fellowships in chemical dependency treatment. Both of these initiatives have furthered the overall aim of the organization of developing some type of specialty or subspecialty status.

American Academy of Psychiatrists in Alcoholism and Addictions (AAPAA)

Founded in 1985, this organization of psychiatrists had grown to 1,029 members as of May 1993. The AAPAA is devoted to upgrading the knowledge and skills of psychiatrists in addiction psychiatry, defining and developing the role of psychiatrists in the treatment system, and improving the quality of patient care. The AAPAA publishes the *American Journal of Addictions* and sponsors an annual scientific meeting. The AAPAA is also concerned with the development of fellowships in chemical dependency and with a variety of practice and policy issues, all from a psychiatric perspective.

Association for Medical Education and Research in Substance Abuse (AMERSA)

AMERSA began in 1976 as an outgrowth of the NIAAA and NIDA Career Teachers program to develop medical school faculty in addiction medicine. AMERSA's 370 members include both physicians and nonphysicians involved in medical education. Its annual meetings and publications focus on educational issues. AMERSA is also active in encouraging the establishment of fellowships in chemical dependency.

Training

Most psychiatrists currently in the field have built upon whatever chemical dependency training was available in their residency programs through reading, attending scientific meetings, taking periodic courses (including the Ruth Fox Course mentioned above), and practicing in clinical settings. In some parts of the country, there are also organized postgraduate training programs available for health care professionals.

In recent years, a small but growing number of clinical fellowships in addiction psychiatry have been established, an effort pioneered by the Veterans Administration. According to Frances and Galanter (1988) and Galanter (1988), a survey of 211 psychiatry residency directors yielded information about 20 established chemical dependency fellowships and 33 programs interested in developing such a fellowship. The authors listed 28 fellowships in operation as of January 1988. Only 8 of these were restricted to psychiatrists.

Until 1997, psychiatrists who wish to become certified by the ABPN as having added qualifications in addiction psychiatry are eligible if they are board certified and have experience in this field. After 1997, psychiatrists will be required to have completed a specialty fellowship in addiction psychiatry before being able to take the examination. Although entrance to the ASAM certification examination does not now require the completion of a fellowship, the ASAM's long-range plans will almost certainly involve the adoption of this requirement as addiction psychiatry moves toward medical subspecialty status. At present, like much else in this field, postgraduate training is in a state of development.

Advantages and Disadvantages of the Field

The choice of the specialty area in which one will work is often a very personal one. Many physicians were originally attracted to medicine because of a personal or family experience with illness, and many found their way into psychiatry for similar reasons. Although—to the best of my knowledge—this issue has not been formally studied, many psychiatrists have observed an apparent overrepresentation of adult children of alcoholic parents in the helping professions, including medicine and psychiatry. Some of my colleagues have chosen the chemical dependency field because of personal experiences, although there are many others, like myself, whose involvement began with interest in a particular patient or treatment method (Blume 1986a).

I have found many personal and professional joys in the treatment of chemically dependent patients. Although these patients may be resistant at times, they begin treatment when they are very sick but during their recovery become very well. Recovered alcoholic and substance-addicted patients and compulsive gamblers who are active in 12-step self-help programs become not only functional but enthusiastic in recovery. They remain in touch, volunteer their time and energy to help those still having difficulties, and have often become good friends. Some decide to change careers after a few years of stable recovery and begin to train as counselors, nurses, psychologists, or social workers. They make excellent treatment team members. The same is true of people from alcoholic or addictive family systems who recover in 12-step programs. The experience of playing a part in these recoveries has been my greatest joy.

It is unfortunate that alcoholism is a familial disease. I have treated children of my older patients, as their own dependence on alcohol or drugs develops, as well as the parents of my younger patients. This can be an interesting experience. I have already mentioned the relationship of chemical dependency to general medicine and the opportunity to work as part of a team and with self-help groups. This team setting also carries the disadvantage of constantly having to explain what I am doing (and why). As a psychodramatist, I have found my brief, postsession staff meetings an excellent forum for teaching psychodynamics. A psychiatrist in this field has endless opportunities to teach.

There are particular advantages for women in the field of addiction psychiatry. The availability of a salaried position with predictable, livable work schedules was lifesaving to me as I raised two children without interrupting my career. One of the other consequences of my gender, I believe, has been my long-standing interest in chemical dependency in women. Women's problems have received relatively little attention in research, outreach, prevention, and treatment in this field until recently (Blume 1986b, 1991a). Chemically dependent women are particularly stigmatized by our society (Blume 1991b) and consequently have severe problems with self-esteem. They are often victims of physical and sexual abuse. Women addicted to alcohol and other chemical substances find a special kind of hope and pride in interacting with a woman psychiatrist.

Minority groups in this country, particularly those who live in poverty and who experience prejudice, have had especially pervasive problems with addictive diseases. African-American, Hispanic, and Native American psychiatrists can be uniquely helpful in prevention, treatment, and research in this field, serving as role models as well as helping professionals. The importance of sociocultural factors in shaping the onset and course of addiction, and in promoting recovery, makes the cross-cultural insights of the international medical graduate a valuable asset.

It is difficult to generalize about income in addiction psychiatry, as work settings are so variable. Employed psychiatrists in this field usually maintain private practices as well. Because of the frequency of legal problems involving alcohol and other drug use, there are many opportunities to act as an expert consultant in both civil and criminal cases. Research and teaching opportunities are also available.

The major disadvantages of the field are related to its relative youth and newcomer status in psychiatry and medicine. Many aspects of the field are still in flux, and plans are still on the drawing board. However, one psychiatrist's uncertainty is another's opportunity to get in on the ground floor.

Conclusion

I have attempted to outline some of the major factors to consider in choosing a psychiatric career in chemical dependency. My point of view is an enthusiastically positive one, as I feel that psychiatrists have a great deal to contribute to this emerging field. It is my fervent hope that the tradition of cooperation with other medical specialties and helping professions will continue to thrive in chemical dependency treatment. The increasing involvement of psychiatrists in the field cannot but contribute toward that goal.

References

Bean-Bayog M, Galanter M, Halikas J, et al: Special report—AMSAODD: plan for certification of members, 1985–1986. Alcohol Clin Exp Res 9:390–392, 1985

Blume SB: Alcoholism, in Current Therapy. Edited by Conn HF. Philadelphia, PA, WB Saunders, 1982, pp 921–924

Blume SB: Psychotherapy in the treatment of alcoholism, in Psychiatry Update: The American Psychiatric Association Annual Review, Vol 3. Edited by Grinspoon L. Washington, DC, American Psychiatric Press, 1984, pp 338–346

Blume SB: Alcoholism rehabilitation: getting involved—a memoir of the 60s, in Alcohol Interventions: Historical and Sociocultural Approaches. Edited by Strug DL, Priyadarsini S, Hyman MM. New York, Haworth Press, 1986a, pp 75–80

Blume SB: Women and alcohol: a review. JAMA 256:1467–1470, 1986b

Blume SB: Sexuality and stigma: the alcoholic woman. Alcohol Health and Research World 15:139–146, 1991a

Blume SB: Women, alcohol and drugs, in A Handbook of Drug and Alcohol Addiction. Edited by Miller NS. New York, Marcel Dekker, 1991b, pp 147–177

Cermak TL: Diagnosing and Treating Codependence. Minneapolis, MN, Johnson Institute Books, 1986

Frances R, Galanter M: Fellowship programs in alcohol and drug abuse. AAPAA Newsletter 3:2, Summer/Fall 1988

Galanter M: Postgraduate certification in alcohol and drug dependence. Alcohol Clin Exp Res 9:387–389, 1985

Galanter M: Postgraduate medical fellowships in alcoholism and drug abuse. New York, New York University, Center for Medical Fellowships in Alcoholism and Drug Abuse, 1988

Helzer JE, Pryzbeck TR: The co-occurrence of alcoholism with other psychiatric disorders in the general population and its impact on treatment. J Stud Alcohol 49:219–224, 1988

Jellinek EM: The Disease Concept of Alcoholism. New Haven, CT, College-University Press, 1960

Meyers JK, Weissman MM, Tischler GL, et al: Six-month prevalence of psychiatric disorders in three communities. Arch Gen Psychiatry 41:959–970, 1984

National Institute on Alcohol Abuse and Alcoholism: Sixth special report to the Congress on alcohol and health (ADM Publ No 87-1519). Washington, DC, U.S. Government Printing Office, 1987

National Institute on Drug Abuse, Division of Epidemiology and Statistical Analysis: Highlights from the 1987 National Drug and Alcoholism Treatment Unit Survey (NDATUS). Rockville, MD, NIDA, 1989

National Institute on Drug Abuse, Division of Epidemiology and Statistical Analysis: Highlights from the 1991 National Drug and Alcoholism Treatment Unit Survey (NDATUS). Rockville, MD, Substance Abuse and Mental Health Services Administration, September 1992

Regier DA, Meyer JK, Kramer LN, et al: The NIMH epidemiological catchment area program. Arch Gen Psychiatry 41:934–941, 1984

Regier DA, Farmer ME, Rae DS, et al: Comorbidity of mental disorders with alcohol and other drug abuse. JAMA 264:2511–2518, 1990

Rinaldi RC, Steindler EM, Wilford BB: Clarification and standardization of substance abuse terminology. JAMA 259:555–557, 1988

Robins LN, Helzer JF, Weissman MM, et al: Lifetime prevalence of specific psychiatric disorders in three sites. Arch Gen Psychiatry 41:949–958, 1984

Russell M, Henderson C, Blume SB: Children of Alcoholics: A Review of the Literature. New York, Children of Alcoholics Foundation, 1985

Zimberg S: The Clinical Management of Alcoholism. New York, Brunner/Mazel, 1982

Section IV:
Practice by Specialty Area

Focus on Specific Treatment Modalities

CHAPTER TWENTY

Psychoanalysis

Malkah T. Notman, M.D.

Psychoanalysis is a scientific discipline first developed by Sigmund Freud in the late 19th century. Freud and Breuer worked with patients suffering from severe hysterical symptoms and discovered that these symptoms could be relieved or would disappear when the patient was able to express verbally the previously unconscious ideas or wishes that were in conflict with values, ideals, and concepts of what was permitted. The conflict between the idea or wish that was forbidden but that pressed for expression and the force that exerted the counterpressure to keep it out of consciousness was understood to produce the symptoms. Hypnosis was originally used as a treatment method but was discarded in favor of a technique that did not require an altered state of consciousness. *Psychoanalysis* developed as a collaborative method involving the relationship between doctor and patient in which the patient told the doctor what was on her or his mind in the form of *free associations*. Resistances to doing so also became the focus of analysis.

Freud's work and that of his colleagues extended to many other kinds of patients and forms of psychopathology. In the early 20th century, he developed a method of dream interpretation that also provided access to the unconscious part of the mind. This method relied on the account of the remembered dream and the exploration of its meaning to the dreamer with the use of free associations and an understanding of the context of the dream and the distortions arising from the process of dreaming.

In recent years, psychoanalysis has been expanded to include the understanding of an individual's development and unconscious conflicts, and also to focus on that person's relationships with others, particularly as these could be understood in the relationship with the analyst (i.e., the transference). Psychoanalysis is considered to be a method of treatment, a theory of the mind and behavior, and a method of exploring mental processes. Psychoanalytic theory is concerned with describing and understanding normal psychological functioning as well as psychopathology.

Description of Psychoanalysis

There are two fundamental underlying hypotheses to psychoanalysis: the principle of *psychic determinism*—that is, the idea that psychological events are not accidental or random, but are determined by those that preceded them—and the proposition that there are many psychic processes that are unconscious (Brenner 1973). These unconscious processes are accessible through an individual's free associations, dreams, and memories, and the exploration of certain of the individual's behaviors. In the process of psychoanalysis, some of the unconscious experiences, memories, and feelings become conscious and, therefore, are more available to become modified. The patient's ways of relating to the analyst and to others can be understood and changed. The person's development and maturation and achievement of gratifications and goals can proceed further. Personality changes as well as symptom relief can take place.

Psychoanalytic theory has changed in many ways since Freud, but the concepts that unconscious mental processes are important and that earlier experiences are significant in understanding current ones are part of all psychoanalytic theories.

As a method of treatment, psychoanalysis depends on a particular kind of therapeutic situation in which the relationship between patient and analyst is central. The patient brings his or her thoughts, fantasies, ideas, and feelings and expresses them verbally to the analyst, who, together with the patient, explores their meaning and emotional connections. The patient relates to the analyst in ways that repeat aspects of significant past relationships. Because these feelings and patterns are "transferred" to the analyst, this phenomenon is called *transference*. The reaction of the analyst to the patient, to some extent determined by the analyst's previous experiences, to some extent by the reality presented by the patient, is called *countertransference*.

Transference and countertransference are part of all relationships. These terms originated in psychoanalysis but have been widely used. Understanding the transference reactions between patient and doctor is very important in medical practice; for example, a patient's attitudes toward authority—whether compliant, rebellious, or confrontational—will be part of his or her reaction to any medical caregiver. Thus, a large part of a patient's responses may arise from the attitudes he or she brings to the situation as habitual responses or may be evoked by the parental or other elements in the relationship.

Because an analyst undergoes personal psychoanalysis as part of his or her training, he or she brings an awareness and understanding of these responses to bear in work with patients. Even if the psychiatrist does not plan to practice psychoanalysis, awareness of these transferential attitudes can be extremely important in any psychiatric practice. Psychoanalysis thus offers training for psychiatrists who are interested in becoming psychoanalysts and also for those who want an in-depth understanding of human behavior with applications for many areas of the field of psychiatry. Psychotherapy, consultations, work with psychosomatic reactions, consultation-liaison work, and many other aspects of psychiatrists' activities are enhanced and enriched by psychoanalytic understanding. In addition, a very valuable function that is served by the personal psychoanalysis that is part of psychoanalytic training is to help the psychiatrist become aware of personal blind spots, understand himself or herself better, and work more effectively with patients, colleagues, and others. A personal analysis obviously can be undertaken without psychoanalytic training. For some psychiatrists, personal psychotherapy can accomplish similar goals, not as extensively, but certainly better than no therapy at all.

Training

Course of Training

Psychoanalytic training takes place as a postgraduate program offered by a psychoanalytic training "institute," which functions like a postgraduate university. One must be accepted for training through an application process similar to that for graduate school admission, a process consisting of an application and interviews.

Psychoanalytic training consists of three parts: personal analysis, usually lasting 4–6 years; course work, extending over 4, 5, or more years, depending on the particular psychoanalytic training institute; and supervised psychoanalytic work, usually with three or four patients. Although there are variations in training approaches, these three components of psychoanalytic training are the essentials that are universally included. Usually one's personal analysis is begun first, then courses follow, and finally supervised psychoanalyses complete the training. Many people complete the courses and continue supervised cases in parallel with other jobs or practice.

Types of Psychoanalytic Institutes

There are many psychoanalytic institutes or training centers in the United States and also several federations or associations of likeminded institutes. The American Psychoanalytic Association has 26 institutes across the country. These institutes are similar in that their theoretical orientation is derived from a classical Freudian orientation, although most institutes now have a much more pluralistic approach and teach other theories as well. Some institutes within the American Psychoanalytic Association have had prominent psychoanalysts and their students who have played an important role, such as Heinz Kohut, in Chicago, who developed the theories of self psychology and the associated modifications in clinical approach. Until very recently, most psychoanalytic institutes affiliated with the American Psychoanalytic Association required a medical degree for full clinical training. Recently, trainees without a medical degree have been admitted to such full training; these are primarily individuals who have completed a doctorate or its equivalent.

Other psychoanalytic institutes following other theoretical orientations (e.g., those following Karen Horney or Carl Jung; the William Alanson White Psychoanalytic School in New York City where Harry Stack Sullivan has been the important theoretical influence) have different approaches; some have admitted trainees with no medical degree—particularly psychologists with a doctorate-level degree—from the beginning. Thus, individuals looking for psychoanalytic training have a choice, both in particular style and in theoretical affiliation of the institute. Currently, all institutes train both psychiatrists and nonmedical specialists.

The particular structure of the psychoanalytic institute varies from place to place, as do universities. Some institutes are closely affiliated with one particular university, as is Columbia University Center for Psychoanalytic Training and Research in New York City, or are loosely affiliated, as is New Orleans Psychoanalytic Institute with Louisiana State University. Others, such as the Boston Psychoanalytic Institute, are not directly affiliated with academic centers although there are many universities in the area and individual candidates and psychoanalysts are affiliated with a variety of academic institutions.

Psychoanalytic training, unlike a fellowship or residency, is not undertaken on a full-time basis. It is generally expected that students or *candidates*, as students are generally called, will work at other jobs and/or be in practice simultaneously with their psychoanalytic training. Seminars usually are held in the evenings or, in some cities where many have to travel long distances to the training center, are grouped around Fridays and Saturdays.

Length of Training

Length of training is somewhat variable, as one important factor is the willingness or the ability of the trainee to see several psychoanalytic patients in supervision simultaneously. For those who do not see their supervised patients all at once, the training period can be quite prolonged, and then becomes just one experience in an otherwise full professional life. Although financial reasons or personal demands, including pregnancy or parenthood, can make for a protracted training period, usually it is most productive to arrange training to be shorter and more intensive. The person who can see supervised cases in an overlapping fashion makes a fairly large commitment to doing psychoanalytic work. Sometimes one must be prepared to see some patients at a lower fee; this is possible if a private practice can balance low-fee cases or if one has other sources of additional financial support.

Essential Skills of a Psychoanalyst

What does it take to be a psychoanalyst? The essential skills are an orientation to, and an interest in, an individual's inner psychological life. Because psychoanalysis is most appropriate for people who are reflective, it takes a capacity for *psychological mindedness*—that is, sensitivity and interest in psychological phenomena, emotional reactions, and states of mind and feeling. Someone who is primarily oriented to action or "fixing" things quickly may not be comfortable with the slow pace and relative lack of action orientation of psychoanalytic work. There are various styles of doing psychoanalytic work, but these basic qualities are always important. It also takes an interest in and capacity to sit with a patient for relatively long periods of time. A psychoanalysis usually lasts for several years and is intensive. The patient is often seen three or four times per week.

Although psychoanalysis itself is only used for treating individuals, psychoanalytic principles and understanding are important in work with groups and families as well. Child psychoanalysis is a subspecialty that requires further training and may involve work with very young children. The child analyst uses play as a means of communicating with the child patient, rather than depending on verbal communication alone.

Financing Psychoanalytic Training

Psychoanalytic training is expensive. Very rarely is there institutional financial support for the actual training.

The most significant expense is one's personal analysis. Tuition for courses is usually comparable with that of any other postgraduate training, and supervision is arranged either as part of tuition or paid for individually as one might pay for private supervision in any setting. Most people finance their psychoanalytic training from earnings from their own practice. In some training centers or departments of psychiatry, the institution lends its support by permitting residents, fellows, faculty, or staff members time off for analysis or supervision hours. On rare occasions, grants may be available for part of the psychoanalytic training.

Patients for supervised psychoanalysis can be obtained in various ways. Most institutes help their candidates arrange for at least the first and often the second patient. In some areas, most psychoanalytic trainees are already in practice, having finished their residencies, and find patients from their own practices.

Current Practice Patterns

Psychoanalysis had a rapid expansion and development after World War II. At that time, most psychiatry department chairs in the United States were psychoanalysts. With the advent of biological psychiatry and with increased understanding of the limitations of psychoanalysis, the popularity of psychoanalysis has diminished. Some have thought that this has its advantages, in that indications for psychoanalysis are more carefully assessed and considered. At the same time, in many training centers there are fewer psychoanalysts and less time devoted to teaching psychoanalytic ideas, so that those who are interested in psychoanalysis have a harder time learning about it, seeing it practiced, or finding practitioners as role models from whom they can learn and with whom they can work. Psychiatry curricula have usually included some psychoanalytic principles, but in some training centers there is not enough clinical teaching to provide an understanding of what is gained by a psychodynamic approach or how it works. Although psychoanalysis is not as popular as it was in the 1960s or 1970s, a significant number of psychiatrists are seeking psychoanalytic training.

Practice styles have also become more variable than they were a generation ago. At that time, there was a tendency for psychoanalysts to be primarily in private practice and to remain somewhat detached from general psychiatry and even more from medicine. Although that is still true for some individuals, the balance has shifted. Most young psychoanalysts today are also involved in other psychiatric or related work; this change will undoubtedly have an effect in integrating their psychoanalytic work into their other fields. Currently, except for some practitioners in larger cities, psychoanalysts usually do not fill their practices exclusively with psychoanalytic patients.

Furthering a Psychoanalytic Career

The career ladder for a psychoanalyst who is primarily working with psychoanalytic patients may include aspirations to be appointed as a training analyst. The term *training analyst* is a designation equivalent to a professorial appointment in an academic setting. Training and supervising analysts are primarily those psychoanalysts who are available for the personal analysis of candidates and for psychoanalytic supervision. They are appointed by institutes after a process of training, review, and some years of experience. The particular procedures and requirements for becoming a training analyst vary from institute to institute, with some requiring more experience than others. Training analysts, by and large, have a larger psychoanalytic practice than other psychoanalysts and participate in teaching, administrative responsibilities, and other academic roles.

Special Issues for Psychoanalysts

Advantages of Psychoanalytic Practice

First, as is true for private practice in general, psychoanalytic practice gives the practitioner the flexibility of setting his or her own work hours. This can be helpful for physicians attempting to balance work and family.

Second, patients who are suitable for psychoanalytic work are by and large less likely to be hospitalized, and less likely to become acutely psychotic or have major crises, as people with severe illnesses tend not to be able to sustain psychoanalytic work.

International Influences in Contemporary Psychoanalysis

A whole generation of psychoanalysts emigrated to the United States from Europe in the 1930s with the advent of Nazism. The popular stereotype of the German-speaking analyst derives not only from Freud and his Viennese background, but also from the prominence of German- and Austrian-trained psychoanalysts who emigrated. American psychoanalysis flourished in the post–World War II era and, for a time, the locus of advances in psychoanalysis shifted from Europe to the United States. It has now again gained momentum in Europe, Japan, and South America. Many of the South American institutes have been strongly influenced by Melanie Klein and to some extent by Jacques Lacan. The International Psychoanalytic Association has acknowledged the multiple theoretical perspectives in contemporary psychoanalysis.

Women and the Practice of Psychoanalysis

Psychoanalysis has always been a field in which women have played an important part. Among Freud's earliest colleagues were Lou-Andreas Salome, Helene Deutsch, Karen Horney, Princess Marie Bonaparte, Grete Bibring, and others. These were all women with an adventurous spirit who differed from their peers, mainly by entering medicine and then psychoanalysis. During the period when very few American women were entering professions, there were still women who were training as psychoanalysts and who became prominent (Chodorow 1990). Marion Kenworthy, Viola Bernard, and Clara Thompson are some of the American women well known for their contributions to American psychoanalysis.

Because the number of women entering medical training did not become significant in the United States until the mid-1970s, their number in psychoanalytic training was limited. The situation has been different for women training in many European countries (e.g., England, France), as well as in a few American institutes, where a medical background has not been required for psychoanalysis; in these situations, the percentage of women in psychoanalytic practice has been higher.

Psychoanalysis is particularly suited to women psychiatrists in several ways. It is primarily a verbal approach, depending on recognition and verbalization of thoughts, fantasies, and wishes, and requires those who are sensitive to emotional states in themselves and others. Women as a group possess these qualities; the orientation to listening and relatively delayed action fits both women with conventional backgrounds and those with nonconventional backgrounds and interests.

In addition, the receptivity of the field to women and the relatively high proportions of women patients add to the suitability of psychoanalysis as a field for women. Many of the past barriers—both internal and external—to women entering psychoanalysis (e.g., the need for medical training) have been removed and women have been entering psychoanalysis in larger numbers. Men continue to occupy many of the positions of leadership and to be attracted to the field as well. The potential flexibility of work hours and office location is compatible with balancing family and work and thus is often a particular advantage for women practitioners.

As more women enter leadership in the field and contribute to the literature, clinical issues and the direction of research are likely to reflect women's concerns more fully.

Freud's formulations about women's development and functioning have been criticized as reflecting views of his phallocentric culture. Modifications of these have already taken place and will continue to take place. Freud's fundamental ideas and their profound importance in describing major determinants of human behavior do not depend on his specific erroneous ideas about women's development and social roles. In taking the complaints and concerns of women seriously in the work on hysteria, he made important contributions. Current and future contributions will continue to modify both theories and formulations as they do in any dynamic field. Many recent theorists have based their work on the fundamental concerns of psychoanalysis with intrapsychic processes, the unconscious, early and later developmental experiences, and the accumulation of clinical experiences and have revised some of the more limited formulations of earlier theorists.

Conclusion

Psychoanalytic training offers a rich experience that deepens understanding and sophistication and prepares psychiatrists for a wide range of further activities. Psychodynamic training provides the psychoanalyst with a fundamental approach to understanding patients, even if other treatment modalities constitute an essential or even primary therapeutic approach.

References

Brenner C: An Elementary Textbook of Psychoanalysis, Revised Edition. Madison, CT, International Universities Press, 1973

Chodorow N: Feminism and psychoanalytic theory, in 70's Questions for 30's Women. New Haven, CT, Yale University Press, 1990, pp 199–218

For Further Reading

Freud S: An outline of psychoanalysis (1938), in The Standard Edition of the Complete Psychological Works of Sigmund Freud, Vol 23. Translated and edited by Strachey J. London, Hogarth Press, 1974, pp 139–171

Menninger K: Theory of Psychoanalytic Technique. New York, Basic Books, 1958

CHAPTER TWENTY-ONE

Family Therapy

Joan J. Zilbach, M.D.

Family therapy had its birth in research in the mid-1950s on families and emerged as a treatment in the 1960s. It occupies an increasing amount of time in the practice of psychiatrists, mental health professionals, and others. However, the "new kid on the block" status attributed to family therapy is evident in many residency training programs, which often still have minimal training opportunities in family work.

There are several indicators of the growth, development, and importance of family therapy, which now has the largest number of practitioners of any mental health field, not only among psychiatrists, psychologists, and social workers, but also among those trained directly in this modality with the professional designation of "marriage and family counselors." Sluzki (1987) described *Family Process*, the first journal in family therapy, as having been "the only tree in places where there now is a forest" of 50 or more family-oriented journals. In addition, the American Association of Marriage and Family Therapists, founded in 1962, is a large and rapidly growing professional organization that certifies supervisors as one of its many functions. The increasing diversity of families and their involvement in psychiatric treatment will also likely continue to grow in the 1990s.

The practice of family therapy itself is but one way psychiatrists work with families. There are family consultations in medical and other settings; "psychoeducation," concerned particularly with families of schizophrenic patients; and family consultations in a variety of institutional systems, including schools, social agencies, corporations, and so forth.

Basics of Family Therapy

Family therapy today exists in many forms, with the universal characteristic of all such therapies being that the family, rather than the individual, is the unit of treatment (Zilbach 1986). The *family* itself requires definition: "A family is a special kind of small, natural group in which members related by birth, marriage, or other form create a home or a functional household unit" (Zilbach 1986, p. 6). This clinically useful definition emphasizes the family as the basic psychosocial unit into which all members are born or inducted by some other means, and emphasizes the primary importance of the family as the operating unit in society. It is a forever-changing and developing unit.

There are many schools of family therapy, which may be broadly categorized as follows:

- Psychoanalytic–object relations family therapy
- Cognitive-behavioral family therapy
- Systemic-strategic family therapy

In all of these therapeutic forms, general systems theory and family systems theory in particular have become the basic underlying theoretical model. All schools teach an understanding of the family as a system within the larger societal context and as a system that contains smaller subgroups of individual members. Thus, a working knowledge of family systems theory is essential for understanding families.

Three basic concepts—*family homeostasis, double-bind communication,* and *family development*—are pillars for understanding families.

- *Family homeostasis*—This concept extends the understanding of homeostatic mechanisms from biology and physiology to psychology and the family. It implies an ever-changing series of alterations in family functions initiated by internal or external changes that result in a return to a form of family stability. This concept is useful in understanding the consistency and stability of family patterns, which may extend over many generations.
- *Double-bind communication*—This concept refers to the simultaneous transmission of contradictory messages in which family

members are caught between two orders of message and are required to respond. Awareness of this family communication pattern is useful in understanding dysfunction or pathology in families (Bateson et al. 1963).
- *Family development*—In contrast to family homeostasis, this concept emphasizes ever-occurring change in families—that is, those changes occurring over time in expectable and observable phases beginning with the birth of the family unit and lasting through its middle and later phases, through its end (Carter and McGoldrick 1980; Zilbach 1986).

Marital or couples treatment is a prevalent subtype of family treatment. When a couple comes to treatment, it is important for the therapist to be able to identify the stage of the family's or couple's development in order to understand the problems or dysfunction with which they present.

The family as a basic psychosocial unit may or may not include children, but when there are children, they deserve particular attention and it is important to include them for a full understanding of the family. In order to include children in family treatment, it is necessary to have basic knowledge of human development and to have simple techniques for comfortably including young family members in family treatment (Zilbach 1986). A good training program should include specific attention to this aspect of family treatment.

Of particular importance are the ethnic and cultural aspects of families, which become an important aspect of family life. At the present, knowledge of Hispanic, African-American, Asian, and other immigrant and ethnic groups is increasingly important for family work in many communities. The family therapist must learn about family cultural contexts by immersion through literature and also in the daily life of such families.

Career Planning in Family Therapy

There are three groups of psychiatrists for whom this orienting sketch of family therapy is relevant: 1) those preparing to enter the field of psychiatry, prior to psychiatric residency; 2) those in psychiatric residency; and 3) those already practicing psychiatry.

- *Prior to psychiatric residency*—Potential psychiatric residents have the opportunity to thoroughly investigate the components of training programs. Three elements require investigation: theory, practice, and supervision. One should find answers to the following questions: Is there a basic course given to residents that encompasses more than one school of family treatment? Are there adequate family cases that include experience with various ethnic groups and with various degrees of dysfunction? Is there adequate and specific supervision by trained and experienced family therapists?
- *Psychiatric residents*—Psychiatrists-in-training may become aware of inadequacies in their family treatment training and may need to search out additional family training experiences.
- *Psychiatrists already in practice*—Working clinicians may become aware of the amount of family work that is clinically indicated or that they are asked to do but for which they are not adequately prepared. There are a number of freestanding family therapy training institutions that may be particularly useful for those already in practice. As these freestanding institutions are evaluated, the same three components of theory instruction, clinical cases, and supervision should be considered.

It is important for students of family therapy to read the literature beyond that of one school of thought (e.g., Papp 1977). In recent years, psychoanalytic–object relations family therapy has become more prominent, but its presentation may be lacking in many present freestanding institutions (see Scharff and Scharff 1987). Another recent element in family therapy has been the influence of gender and feminist considerations (see Luepnitz 1988).

Residents often participate in individual psychotherapy in the course of residency, and in addition, many residencies have didactic training groups that are useful both personally and in group therapy work. However, most trainees do not have the opportunity to explore the impact of family on themselves and their families and tend to rely on techniques for family work derived from their experience with individual psychodynamic psychotherapy, whether as patients or practitioners. Some training institutions meet this need with a specifically designed family training group (Bennett and Zilbach 1989), whereas others have "family of origin" groups (Kramer 1989). Many institutions do not meet this need, but it is important for those embarking on family training to realize that there will be considerable impact on their understanding and feelings about their own families.

Conclusion

In *Anna Karenina,* Tolstoy wrote, "All happy families resemble one another; every unhappy family is unhappy in its own way." The emergence of family therapy as a treatment modality, and family systems theory as a model for understanding families, may help practitioners understand how happy families resemble one another and how to assist unhappy families in surmounting the challenges and the dysfunctions of their family lives. Family therapy has grown rapidly into many schools of treatment, but there are underlying principles that form the basis for family therapy as a field. As mentioned previously, working with families is likely to occupy a growing amount of psychiatric practice, and, therefore, training opportunities need to be both developed and expanded. The basic information in this chapter may assist people entering the field, in the field, and in practice to acquire knowledge or to upgrade their knowledge of families in many forms and in many stages of the family life cycle.

References

Bateson G, Jackson DD, Haley J, et al: A note on the double bind. Fam Process 2:154–161, 1963
Bennett MI, Zilbach JJ: An experiential family therapy training seminar, in Children in Family Therapy: Treatment and Training. Edited by Zilbach JJ. New York, Haworth Press, 1989, pp 145–155
Carter E, McGoldrick M (eds): The Family Life Cycle: A Framework for Family Therapy. New York, Gardner Press, 1980

Kramer JR: Perceived change in self and children following participation of a therapist-parent in a therapist's own family group, in Children in Family Therapy: Treatment and Training. Edited by Zilbach JJ. New York, Haworth Press, 1989, pp 173–184

Luepnitz D: The Family Interpreted: Feminist Theory in Clinical Practice. New York, Basic Books, 1988

Papp P: Family Therapy: Full Length Case Studies. New York, Gardner Press, 1977

Scharff D, Scharff J: Object Relations Family Therapy. Northvale, NJ, Jason Aronson, 1987

Sluzki CE: Family process: mapping the journey over twenty-five years. Fam Process 26(2):149–152, 1987

Zilbach JJ: Young Children in Family Therapy. New York, Brunner/Mazel, 1986

For Further Reading

Bertallanffy von L: General Systems Theory. New York, Braziller, 1968

Guerin PJ: Family therapy: the first twenty-five years, in Family Therapy: Theory and Practice. Edited by Guerin PJ. New York, Gardner Press, 1976, pp 2–23

Gurman AS, Kniskern DP: Handbook of Family Therapy. New York, Brunner/Mazel, 1981

Hoffman L: Foundations of Family Therapy. New York, Basic Books, 1981

Zilbach JJ: Children in Family Therapy: Treatment and Training. New York, Haworth Press, 1989

CHAPTER TWENTY-TWO

Group Therapy

Marcia Slomowitz, M.D.

The Basis for Group Therapy

Most human beings live their lives in groups. Born and usually raised in families, children have an infinite number of interactions with mother, father, grandparents, siblings, and other extended family members. Beyond the boundary of the family, children go to school, where they develop peer groups as their own social networks. In adolescence, these social ties assume a prime position. Adults who wish to recreate the comfort of their earlier family environment move toward creation of a new nuclear family. At the same time, they frequently work in an organized setting. Individuals also consider themselves members of groups by gender, race, ethnicity, age, religion, marital status, socioeconomic status, and occupation. As people live their lives with the accompanying developmental vicissitudes, participation in such groups evolves. Joining, establishing oneself in, and leaving the respective groups can both create psychological dilemmas and expose existing vulnerabilities, as issues of intimacy and individuation constantly resurface.

Certain larger cultural forces affect the psychological readiness of people to commit to a group, influencing how they feel about themselves and others. Specific factors—for example, breakdown of the extended (and often the nuclear) family, enhanced geographic mobility, and changing roles of women—have been considered as leading to a generalized loss of the expectation of stability and an increased incidence of depression (Klerman and Weissman 1989).

The capacity to engage in and maintain interpersonal relationships and to be intimate is severely tested with these social realities. It is not surprising, therefore, that many authors have described changes they have seen in clinical practice with regard to individual psychopathology, noting especially an increase in narcissistic and borderline issues, in which one's capacity for intimate human relationships is severely disabled. Group therapy has been described as the "natural antidote" to these disorders commonly encountered in clinical work and, as such, is an obvious treatment modality for psychiatrists to practice (Rutan and Stone 1984).

Patient Population and Process

Psychiatrists with group psychotherapy training have at their disposal a treatment modality applicable to a variety of settings and patient populations. Patients can be seen in a private outpatient practice with group therapy as the primary modality of treatment, or in conjoint treatment with individual psychotherapy (Day 1970; Ormont 1981). Group treatment of patients on short-term inpatient units has also been described (Kibel 1981; Yalom 1983). In addition, groups have been recommended as the treatment of choice for adolescents (Rutan and Stone 1984).

Regardless of the setting or composition of the group, a benefit of group psychotherapy is the opportunity for both patient and clinician to see behavior that can only be described secondhand in individual psychotherapy. A patient's complaint of being unable to develop or maintain intimate relationships will be more clearly understood as that person interacts with other group members and the therapist.

One frequently occurring phenomenon in groups illustrating such actions or behaviors is *scapegoating*. In this scenario, feelings and attitudes members do not consciously want to attribute to themselves are projected onto a victim. The work of the group allows individuals to discover and reclaim their projections, then to understand and own them. For the other group members, too, scapegoating offers the opportunity to learn which of their behaviors may have contributed to being the chosen target (Rutan and Stone 1984).

The psychological mechanisms responsible for change in individuals in group psychotherapy have been listed as imitation, identification, and internalization (Rutan and Stone 1984). In group settings, members have the possibility of watching many different kinds of interactions among individuals. As a precursor to more intimate relationships involving more personal sharing of feelings, the group setting allows a person to observe how others go about revealing feelings. *Imitation* can lead to enhanced competence and self-confidence. At another level, *identification* forms a basis for more lasting psychological change. This unconscious process, in which individuals *internalize* parts of other individuals, members, and therapists, facilitates changes in how participants respond to one another. Identification, the most permanent of the mechanisms, results from a shift in psychic structure and can be observed in group members as they engage in new behavior and recognize the changes in the way they act.

The therapeutic processes through which internalizations, including identification and imitation, occur are enriched in a group setting. *Confrontation* (i.e., the noting of specific behavior in one individual by another) has multiple potential participants. Confrontations may come from one or more members as well as from the therapist; of course, in individual psychotherapy, this is the therapist's job alone. Both the ability to confront another person and the capacity to reflect on having been confronted are frequent psychotherapy treatment goals. The act of confrontation in a group encourages the development of empathy with the feelings of other members. *Clarification* also has a wider arena for use in group therapy than in individual treatment, as the group as a whole provides a richer source of experiences for group members to draw upon. *Interpretation* (i.e., making the unconscious conscious) is also enhanced in a group, as group experience provides fertile ground for affect needed to take in an interpretation.

Confrontation, clarification, and interpretation may lead to narcissistic injury, allowing the opportunity to scrutinize the process that led to the narcissistic imbalance. The "working through" process of repair is enhanced by the group experience. Multiple and repeated here-and-now interactions with group members lead to immediate feedback. The process of reparation of the narcissistic injury occurs along with a shift in defensive structure. Outside events are discussed with the hope that this process will ultimately lead to an enhanced cognitive understanding of behavior. The group experiences repetitive events and multiple relationships with opportunities to practice new ways to cope with anxieties.

Although the above descriptions are of group psychotherapy as a vehicle for psychological change, group psychotherapy may also have the tasks of stabilization of psychotic states and maintenance or improvement of affective relationships in the treatment of more severely impaired, chronically mentally ill patients. The work may be more concrete and may include assistance in living with persistent auditory hallucinations and assessment of need for and benefit from medication. Even with this more disabled patient population, group therapy can provide valuable aid in rehabilitation and socialization.

An additional benefit for all patients in group treatment is the financial one. In comparison with individual psychotherapy, the fees charged per person in group psychotherapy are substantially lower, generally with increased revenue per clinician hour for the individual therapist or the agency. Given current trends to reduce health care costs by third-party payers and to expand health maintenance organizations and other managed care systems, group psychotherapy will likely become a more popular treatment modality.

Training

Recognition of the need for psychiatrists to acquire skills as group therapists is exemplified by the results of a recent study examining education for residents. In a survey of American psychiatric residency programs, 78% of those responding offered group psychotherapy training (Pinney et al. 1978). Sixty-two percent of the programs offered such work over 3–4 postgraduate years, with the predominant teaching methods being didactic, experiential groups, and supervision. Thus, group psychotherapy training is widely accepted in psychiatric residency training programs.

Training in group psychotherapy with the concomitant focus on group dynamics gives psychiatrists comfort in addressing systems issues. They gain expertise in providing consultation in complex intraprofessional and interdisciplinary arenas. Clearly, with the ever-expanding role of managed care, it is imperative that psychiatrists maintain administrative acumen in sorting out inevitable clinical, ethical, and economic conflicts.

Working with colleagues on patient care involves a knowledge of systems issues. As Astrachan (1970) pointed out,

> without an appreciation of the impact of the structure of the therapy on patient behavior, the temptation is to perceive the patient's behavior as individually determined, be it conscious or unconscious, and to ignore the manner in which the setting facilitates or inhibits feelings and actions. (p. 114)

This concept has long been understood in relation to patients on inpatient units; however, it is equally true in other settings. Before the meaning of a patient's symptoms or behavior can be understood, the environment in which the patient lives must be studied. For example, a patient's symptoms may be a reflection of underlying tensions between staff members or a result of misdirected communications (Stanton and Schwartz 1954). Psychiatrists who have an appreciation of these issues and the ability to use systems thinking will find that their skills are valuable in work with patients and are sought out by colleagues.

Special Issues

Lack of exclusivity for psychiatrists. One key dilemma for psychiatrists is that being a group psychotherapist does not coincide with their primary professional identity. Psychiatrists may consider that they have expertise with particular patient populations or in certain settings. As with other psychotherapies, doing group psychotherapy is a skill for which other disciplines have training, contributing to the lack of central identity for psychiatrists. There are no national organizations of group psychotherapists who are psychiatrists only. In an attempt to counteract this identity diffusion, regional and national organizations sponsor educational meetings both to improve skills and to enhance camaraderie among group psychotherapists. The American Psychiatric Association and the American Group Psychotherapy Association both recognize this problem and are developing links between the two organizations to decrease isolation between psychiatrists doing group psychotherapy.

Second-class status among psychotherapeutic modalities. Despite the fact that a significant number of American psychiatric residency programs offer training in group psychotherapy, concerns have been raised about the quality of that training. In part, this seems to stem from the second-class status group therapy has as a treatment choice, and the fact that it is often used only as a matter of expediency (Johnson and Howenstine 1982). Poor training may reflect the lack of availability of highly trained psychiatrists with group therapy skills, interests, and enthusiasm.

This all-too-common second-class status of group psychotherapy contributes to group psychiatrists' identity issues. In a recent study of an institution that wished to enhance the status of group psychotherapy, three factors were identified as contributing to this scenario (Johnson and Howenstine 1982). First, the cultural emphasis on individualism leads to the frequent choice of individual psychotherapy over all other treatment modalities. Second, the fear of conducting group psychotherapy by new group therapy trainees and residents was noted. Therapists cannot hide in a group; thus, groups heighten their anxiety about revealing ignorance or inadequacy. Although many therapists learn about individual psychotherapy from their own treatment experience, group therapists seldom have this opportunity. Lack of available psychotherapy groups, anxiety over joining a group, and the cultural preference for individual work make this experience less likely. Third, the low academic status of group psychotherapy was noted. Whereas a literature on group psychotherapy does exist, it is markedly smaller than the body of writings on other psychotherapies. This observation reinforces the second-class status of group psychotherapy.

Group psychotherapy used as a last resort. Group psychotherapy referrals are frequently made when no other treatment is available. As such, clinicians feel that they are referring patients to second-class treatment. Although there are guidelines for the selection of patients for group psychotherapy and for assessing appropriateness of fit between patient and group, this information is not frequently used by therapists in determining the appropriate mode of treatment (Grunebaum and Kates 1977).

Conclusion

Clearly, advocacy of group psychotherapy must occur at the highest administrative and educational levels. Psychiatrists are in a unique position to encourage the development of group psychotherapy treatment, training, and research programs, as they can authorize the legitimacy of the program and the group leaders and allocate needed resources. A core of committed psychiatrists will spawn future group psychotherapists whose skills will be valued in the coming years. Studies of the efficacy and outcome of different models of group treatment for different patient populations are needed. Psychiatrists can provide leadership in doing or facilitating group therapy research to enhance its academic status.

In a more controlled health care system, group psychotherapy training will enhance psychiatrists' ability to understand and treat patients who are more disturbed. It behooves psychiatrists to use these group skills and their professional status in dealing most effectively with the psychological, social, biological, and economic problems of the 1990s.

References

Astrachan BM: Towards a social systems model of therapeutic groups. Social Psychiatry 5:110–119, 1970

Day M: Psychoanalytic group therapy in clinic and private practice. Am J Psychiatry 138:64–79, 1970

Grunebaum H, Kates W: Whom to refer for group psychotherapy. Am J Psychiatry 134:130–133, 1977

Johnson D, Howenstine R: Revitalizing an ailing group psychotherapy program. Psychiatry 45:138–146, 1982

Kibel HD: A conceptual model for short-term inpatient group psychotherapy. Am J Psychiatry 138:74–80, 1981

Ormont LR: Principles and practice of conjoint psychoanalytic treatment. Am J Psychiatry 138:69–74, 1981

Pinney EL, Wells SH, Fisher B: Group therapy training in psychiatric residency programs: a national survey. Am J Psychiatry 135:1505–1508, 1978

Rutan JS, Stone WN: Psychodynamic Group Psychotherapy. Lexington, MA, DC Heath, 1984

Stanton AH, Schwartz MS: The Mental Hospital. New York, Basic Books, 1954

Yalom ID: Inpatient Group Psychotherapy. New York, Basic Books, 1983

Conclusion

Leah J. Dickstein, M.D.
Kathleen M. Mogul, M.D.

As we write this conclusion, it is now early 1995. The book has taken considerable time to write, rewrite, update, and edit; even so, there have probably been changes since chapters were last rewritten, and further ones may occur before the publication date in a few months.

The national and congressional health care debate of the last year, together with the effective advocacy of organized psychiatry—led by the American Psychiatric Association (APA)—and patient and family advocacy groups has resulted in raised public awareness of the need for insurance to cover mental health care. Most bills under consideration in the summer of 1994 included more generous and even more equitable coverage than is now generally available. The failure of health care legislation in the early autumn of 1994 signals that major problems in health care will continue for those who need it and those who provide it. The number of Americans who are uninsured increased in 1993 by 1.1 million to 39.7 million, or 15.3% of the population.

Whereas our prediction that universal health care might be enacted by Congress has not come true, the prediction that the penetration by managed care would increase has been borne out. Various innovative treatment approaches are receiving financial support in the attempt to avert more costly hospitalization. There is increasing interference by managers of care with hospitalization of patients by clinicians; length of hospital stays are controlled by managers and are becoming shorter and shorter. There is no reliable information to evaluate the comparative quality of these newer treatment approaches.

Although many psychiatrists see mainly intrusion and problems arising from managed systems of care, others are adapting their way of practice and using new approaches; still others find challenge or opportunity in becoming the managers of care or the developers of criteria for treating patients as economically as possible. There is general agreement that guidelines for diagnostic procedures and treatment for various conditions need to be developed (and the APA and other organizations are doing this), and that outcome evaluations that use multiple criteria (e.g., from patient satisfaction to number of hospitalizations and relapse rates) to compare different approaches are needed.

What has not changed and will not change is our patients' great need both for understanding and for informed and up-to-date care and treatment. Likewise unchanging is the tremendous challenge for psychiatrists in research, administrative, and clinical fields to provide effective services and to make new discoveries that enlarge what we know and lead ultimately to ever-improving treatment for patients with psychiatric disorders.

The authors of this book have offered clear introductions to various ways of practicing psychiatry and have conveyed the challenges, knowledge, and satisfactions to be found, now as always, within this medical specialty. They have also given practical details about training, the effect of work on lifestyle, and other considerations that go into career decisions and planning. In combination with information from experienced colleagues, from training program brochures and training directors, this book should provide a useful guide for making career decisions.

Our commitment to address within each chapter the special advantages and problems for women and minority psychiatrists highlights those issues that continue to challenge members of these groups in many settings. These remarks are meant to help them and their concerned colleagues to confront relevant issues forthrightly. We encourage medical students, residents, faculty, and staff in all professional arenas to advocate for parental leave and dependent care provisions, as well as for other benefits, such as flexible working conditions and supports, that will allow all psychiatrists—women and men alike—to enjoy successful, satisfying personal lives as they pursue vocational goals throughout their professional careers.

As this Decade of the Brain reaches its halfway mark, scientific knowledge of the human mind, brain, and body and of their connections continues to increase at an exponential rate. Indeed, throughout our own decades of experience as psychiatrists, we and our colleagues have experienced the excitement of watching these advances in understanding lead to more humane and effective options for diagnosing and treating those suffering from psychiatric illness. We have seen these improved approaches and treatments yield returns of considerable value—the alleviation of pain and distress in the individuals who seek our help. Witnessing and participating in our patients' remarkable improvements and recoveries is a great privilege that amply rewards our commitment and efforts. We urge you, the reader, to discover these challenges and satisfactions for yourself.

Index

Academic psychiatry
  accreditation of as specialty, 176–179
  administration and, 171–172
  benefits and difficulties of career in, 164–165
  career opportunities in, 157–161
  research and, 163–164
  social issues in, 165–166
  teaching and, 161–163
Academy of Psychosomatic Medicine, 80
Accreditation. *See* Certification
Accreditation Council for Graduate Medical Education, 189
Addiction psychiatry. *See also* Alcoholism
  advantages and disadvantages of careers in, 235–237
  chemical dependency treatment system, 230–232
  establishment of as specialty, 228–229
  growth of treatment system, 232–233
  history of, 229–230
  professional organizations in, 233–235
  training for, 235

Administration. *See also* Administrative psychiatry; Management skills
  academic psychiatry and, 159–160
  definition of, 177
  geriatric psychiatry and, 205
  military psychiatry and, 148
  perceptions of by psychiatrists, 171–172
  of private practices, 96–97
Administrative psychiatry. *See also* Administration
  benefits of careers in, 180
  characteristics of effective administrators, 173–174
  education and training for, 174–176
  special populations and, 179–180
Administration on Aging, 206
Advertising, of private practices, 99
Age. *See also* Elderly; Geriatric psychiatry
  ageism and geriatric psychiatry, 199–200
  increase in elderly population, 62, 198
AIDS (acquired immunodeficiency syndrome)
  child psychiatry and, 186

273

AIDS *(continued)*
  community psychiatrists and, 137
  inpatient psychiatrists and, 62
Alcoholics Anonymous, 229
Alcoholism. *See also* Addiction psychiatry
  dual diagnoses and, 227–228
  family dynamics in, 228
  prevalence of, 227
American Academy of Psychiatrists in Alcoholism and Addictions (AAPAA), 234
American Academy of Child and Adolescent Psychiatry (AACAP), 186, 190, 192, 193
American Association for Geriatric Psychiatry (AAGP), 205–206, 208
American Association of Community Psychiatrists (AACP), 133–134, 140
American Association of Emergency Psychiatrists, 72
American Association of Marriage and Family Therapists, 255
American Board of Psychiatry and Neurology (ABPN), 73, 176, 202–203, 229
American College Health Association, 120
American College of Psychiatrists' Psychiatric Residents-in-Training Examination, 73
American Group Psychotherapy Association, 265
American Journal of Addictions, 234
American Medical Association (AMA)
  Accreditation Council for Graduate Medical Education, 42
  Current Procedural Terminology codes for evaluation/management, 200
  House of Delegates, 193, 230
  practice parameters, development by, 92
American Medical Women's Association (AMWA), 100
American Orthopsychiatric Association, 186
American Psychiatric Association (APA)
  advocacy of organized psychiatry, 269
  annual meeting of, 160
  certification in administrative psychiatry, 176
  Committee on Occupational Psychiatry, 104
  Council on Aging, 205, 206
  group therapy and, 265

Index

practice parameters, development by, 92
Psychiatric Knowledge and Skills Assessment Program, 73
research training and, 13–14
Task Force on Psychiatric Emergency Care Issues, 66, 72–73
American Psychiatric Association Directory of Psychiatry Residency Programs, 175
American Psychoanalytic Association, 246
American Sleep Disorders Association (ASDA), 43
American Society of Addiction Medicine (ASAM), 229–230, 233–234
Apprenticeship model, of research training, 12
Association for Medical Education and Research in Substance Abuse (AMERSA), 234–235
Association of Polysomnographic Technologists (APT), 43
Association of Professional Sleep Societies (APSS), 42–43
Association of Sleep Disorders Centers (ASDC), 36
Association for the Study of Dreams, 43

Behavioral sciences, career opportunities in research, 3–4
Burnout
community psychiatry and, 136
consultation-liaison psychiatry and, 79, 80
inpatient psychiatry and, 54

Canada, residency programs in geriatric psychiatry, 198
Capitation fees, 125
Careers in
academic psychiatry, 157–167
addiction psychiatry, 227–238
administrative psychiatry, 171–180
child psychiatry, 185–194
community psychiatry, 133–140
consultation-liaison psychiatry, 77–86
educational psychiatry, 113–122
family therapy, 255–259
forensic psychiatry, 211–224
geriatric psychiatry, 197–208
group therapy, 261–267
health maintenance organization psychiatry, 125–131
inpatient psychiatry, 51–62
military psychiatry, 143–153
occupational psychiatry, 103–110

Careers in *(continued)*
  private practice, 91–101
  psychiatric research, 3–14, 17–24
  psychoanalysis, 243–252
  psychopharmacology, 25–33
  sleep disorders medicine, 35–45
Caregivers, of elderly, 199, 207
Carve-out arrangements, 125
Certification
  of addiction psychiatry as specialty, 229, 234, 235
  of administrative psychiatry as specialty, 176–179
  in child psychiatry, 189
  in forensic psychiatry, 214–215
  in geriatric psychiatry, 202–203
  in sleep medicine, 42
Chief residency, 175
Child psychiatry
  economics of, 190–191
  ethics in, 192
  history of, 185–186
  legal issues in, 191–192
  psychoanalysis and, 248
  research in, 189–190
  scope of, 186–187
  skills required for, 187–188
  special opportunities and problems in, 192–194
  training for, 189
  work settings in, 188
Children of Alcoholics Foundation, 228

Civil law, forensic psychiatry and, 215–217
Codependence, alcoholism and, 228
Colleges. *See* Academic psychiatry; Educational psychiatry
Commitment law, forensic psychiatry and, 220
Committees, assignments to in academic psychiatry, 160
Community
  private practice and volunteer work in, 100
  role of psychiatrist in military, 145–148
Community hospitals, private practitioners as staff members, 99–100
Community mental health centers, psychiatry in
  career opportunities in, 134–135
  characteristics required for careers in, 139–140
  community psychiatry movement and, 52–53
  current initiatives in, 137–139
  emergency psychiatry and, 65–66
  history of, 133–134
  personal considerations in, 136–137
  psychopharmacology in, 28
  role of psychiatrists in, 135–136

Community Mental Health
  Centers Act (1963), 52, 140
Competency, forensic
  psychiatry and evaluation
  of, 216–217, 218, 219–220
Confidentiality
  in educational psychiatry,
    118–119
  in military psychiatry, 152
  in private practice, 92, 98
Consultation-liaison psychiatry
  career opportunities in, 81–
    82
  child psychiatry and, 188
  educational psychiatry and,
    117–118
  emergency psychiatry and, 72
  forensic psychiatry and, 221–
    222
  geriatric psychiatry and, 203
  history of, 77–78
  legal issues in, 82
  medical specialties and, 82–
    86
  military psychiatry and, 147–
    148
  nature of practice in, 78–80
  occupational psychiatry and,
    106–107
  training in, 80–81
Council for Graduate Medical
  Education, 203
Counselors, chemical
  dependency, 230–231
Countertransference
  educational psychiatry and,
    118

psychoanalysis and, 245
Couples therapy, 257
Court system. *See* Forensic
  psychiatry; Legal issues
Criminal law, forensic
  psychiatry and, 218–220
*Current Procedural Termin-
  ology* (AMA 1992), 200
Curriculum, for occupational
  psychiatry, 110
Custody litigation, forensic
  psychiatry and, 217–218

Daytime sleepiness, 37
Death penalty, forensic
  psychiatry and, 219–220
Deinstitutionalization, 52–53
Delirium, 79
Dementia, 62
Developmental process,
  research training as, 13
Diagnosis
  emergency psychiatry and, 70
  inpatient psychiatry and, 60
Disability, forensic psychiatry
  and evaluation of, 216
Divorce
  dream experience and adapta-
    tion to, 37–38
  forensic psychiatry and litiga-
    tion on, 217
Double-bind communication,
  256–257
Dreaming, sleep disorders and,
  35, 36, 37–38
Drug abuse, prevalence, 227.
  See also Addiction psychiatry

Economics. *See also* Funding; Income
  of child psychiatry, 190–191
  of military psychiatry, 149–150
  of private practice, 91–92
  of psychopharmacology, 31–32
  of somnology, 43–44
Education. *See also* Teaching; Training programs
  forensic psychiatry and public, 224
  in sleep disorders medicine, 41–42
Educational psychiatry
  career opportunities in, 119–121
  financial and practical considerations in, 121
  future of, 122
  history of, 113–114
  legal issues in, 119
  patient population at Student Mental Health Services, 114–116
  roles of student health psychiatrist, 117–118
  special considerations in, 118–119
Elderly. *See also* Geriatric psychiatry
  increase in population of, 62, 198
  poverty and, 207
  problems with delivery of care to, 198–201

Emergency psychiatry
  challenges of, 68–71
  description of, 67
  history of, 65–66
  legal issues in, 74
  nature of, 66–67
  opportunities in and responsibilities of, 72–73
  training programs for, 71–72
  work conditions in, 67–68
Employee assistance programs (EAPs), 108
Ethics. *See also* Values
  administrative psychiatry and, 177
  child psychiatry and, 192
  military psychiatry and, 151–152
  of psychiatrist-researcher, 9
Ethnicity. *See* Minorities
Evaluation and management codes (Medicare), 200–201
Executive directors, of community mental health centers, 135

Family. *See also* Family therapy
  alcoholism and dynamics of, 228
  basic concepts of, 256–257
  definition of, 256
  emergency psychiatry and crises in, 70
Family Process, 255
Family therapy
  basics of, 256–257
  career planning in, 257–259

history of, 255
Fees. *See also* Economics;
    Income
  average in private practice, 93
  Medicare evaluation and
    management codes,
    200–201
Fiscal management,
    administrative psychiatry
    and, 177
Forensic psychiatry
  areas of interest in, 215–223
  challenges in, 223–224
  child psychiatry and, 191–
    192
  criteria for and training as,
    214–215
  definition and history of,
    211–213
  geriatric psychiatry and, 203–
    204
Funding
  for community psychiatry
    programs, 138
  for research, 4–5, 232
  of training programs in geriatric psychiatry, 202

General hospitals, inpatient psychiatry in, 55–56
Geographic location, of new
    private practices, 97–98
Geriatric psychiatry
  description of, 197–198
  and future of inpatient psychiatry, 62
  history of, 197

  problems with delivery of
    care to elderly, 198–201
  professional organizations
    for, 205–206
  special issues in, 206–208
  training programs in, 201–
    203
  work settings in, 203–205
Government, federal, funding
    of psychiatric research, 4–5
Grants, applications for
    research, 7–8
Group for the Advancement of
    Psychiatry (GAP), 104
Group therapy
  basis for, 261–262
  future of, 267
  patient population and process of, 262–264
  special issues in, 265–266
  training for, 264–265
"Guidelines for Psychiatric
    Practice in Staff Model
    HMOs" (APA), 130–131,
    139
Gynecology, consultation
    psychiatry and, 83–86

Health care system. *See also*
    Health maintenance organizations; Insurance, health;
    Managed care
  current crisis in, 269
  occupational psychiatry and,
    108
  recent changes in private
    practice, 91–92

Health maintenance
   organizations, psychiatry in
   career opportunities in, 126–
      127
   clinical practice and, 128–129
   fundamental conflict in, 127–
      128
   history of, 125–126
   psychiatrists as employees,
      129–130
   skills required for work in,
      130–131
Homeless, mentally ill persons
   as, 53
Home office, for private
   practice, 98
Homosexuality
   educational psychiatry and,
      115
   military psychiatry and, 152–
      153

Income. *See also* Economics;
   Fees
   of emergency psychiatrists,
      68
   in private practice, 93
Informed consent, 32
Inpatient psychiatry
   administrative duties in,
      172
   advantages and disadvan-
      tages of careers in,
      53–55
   different settings for, 55–60
   emergency psychiatry and, 73
   future of, 61–62

   history of, 51–53
   prerequisites for, 60–61
   private practice combined
      with, 98–99
   special considerations in,
      61
Insanity defense, forensic
   psychiatry and, 212,
   218–219
Insomnia, 37
Insurance, health. *See also*
   Health maintenance
   organizations; Managed
   care
   educational psychiatry and,
      121
   elderly individuals and geriat-
      ric psychiatry, 201
   health care crisis and, 269
   private practice and, 96, 97
Intentional torts, 216
International medical graduates
   (IMGs), in administrative
   psychiatry. *See also*
   Minorities
International Psychoanalytic
   Association, 251

Joint Commission on the Ac-
   creditation of Healthcare
   Organizations, 73
Journal of Addictive Diseases,
   234
*Journal of American College
   Health,* 120
Journals, family-oriented, 255.
   See also Literature

Juvenile criminal cases, forensic psychiatry and, 220

Lecturing, in preclinical psychiatry, 161–163
Legal issues. *See also* Forensic psychiatry
  in administrative psychiatry, 177
  in child psychiatry, 191–192
  in consultation-liaison psychiatry, 82
  in educational psychiatry, 119
  in emergency psychiatry, 74
  in inpatient psychiatry, 60
  in psychopharmacology, 32
  in sleep disorders medicine, 44–45
Literature, on occupational psychiatry, 106, 110

Malpractice litigation, forensic psychiatry and, 216
Managed care. *See also* Health care system; Health maintenance organizations; Insurance, health
  inpatient psychiatry and, 54–55
  private practice and, 99
  role of psychiatrist in, 269–270
Management skills, required for careers in research, 7–8. *See also* Administration
Marital therapy, 257
Marketing, of private practices, 99
Medical Corps. *See* Military psychiatry
Medical schools, academic psychiatry and teaching in, 161–163
Medicare, geriatric psychiatry and, 199–201, 204
Medigap, 201
Mental hospitals. *See also* Community hospitals; State hospitals
  history of, 51–53
  inpatient psychiatry in, 58
Mentor, role of in research training, 10–11
Methadone treatment clinics, 232
Military psychiatry
  career issues in, 148–150
  description of, 143–145
  ethical considerations in, 151–152
  in the 1990s, 152–153
  role of psychiatrist in military community, 145–148
  training for, 150
  women and minorities in, 151
Minorities, racial and ethnic
  academic psychiatry and, 165
  addiction psychiatry and, 237
  administrative psychiatry and, 179–180
  child psychiatry and, 193
  geriatric psychiatry and, 207
  military psychiatry and, 151

Mobile crisis teams, in community psychiatric programs, 137
Molecular biology, 18
Motives, of psychiatrist-researcher, 9
Multidisciplinary teams
  geriatric psychiatry and, 204–205
  inpatient psychiatry and, 60–61
  psychopharmacology and, 28–29

National Alliance for the Mentally Ill, 134
National Council on Alcoholism and Drug Dependence, 229
National Institute on Aging, 206
National Institute of Mental Health (NIMH), 4–5, 29, 205, 206
Natural disasters, military psychiatrists and, 148
Neuroscience
  career opportunities in research, 3
  and history of psychopharmacology, 26–27
Nursing homes, geriatric psychiatry in, 204

Obstetrics-gynecology, consultation psychiatry and, 83–86

Occupational psychiatry
  career opportunities in, 105–107
  future of, 107–109
  history of, 103–105
  training programs in, 109–110
Office setting, of private practice, 98
On-site supervision, in emergency psychiatry, 72

Patient-centered consultation, as model of psychiatric consultation, 78
Patient population
  in consultation-liaison psychiatry, 79
  in educational psychiatry, 114–116, 119–120
  in emergency psychiatry, 68
  for group therapy, 262–264
  in private practice, 98
  training programs in psychopharmacology and, 30–31
Patient rights, forensic psychiatry and, 220–221
Pediatrics, as medical specialty, 185
Peer reviewers, of research grants, 7–8
Personal injury litigation, 215
Ph.D. model, of research training, 12
Polysomnography, 39
Postresidency fellowships, 175

Posttraumatic stress disorder (PTSD), 215
Poverty, elderly individuals and, 207
Preferred provider organizations (PPOs), 125. *See also* Health maintenance organizations
Preventive health case, and consultation psychiatry, 83–84
Prisons, forensic psychiatry in, 221–222, 224
Private hospitals, inpatient psychiatry in, 58–59
Private practice
    academic psychiatry and, 160–161
    advantages of, 94–95
    characteristics of, 93–94
    consultation psychiatry and, 82
    current data on patterns in, 93
    drawbacks of, 95–97
    economics of, 91–92
    psychopharmacology in, 28
    starting of career in, 97–100
    supports for, 100–101
Professional organizations
    for academic psychiatry, 160
    for addiction psychiatry, 233–235
    for administrative psychiatry, 179
    for child psychiatry, 193
    for geriatric psychiatry, 205–206
    for group therapy, 265
    for occupational psychiatry, 105
    for private practice, 100
    for sleep disorders medicine, 42–43
Psychiatric Research Report (APA), 14
Psychiatric emergency, definition of, 66
Psychiatric Research Resource Center (APA), 14
Psychoanalysis
    career ladder for, 250
    child psychiatry and, 186
    current practice patterns in, 249
    description of, 244–245
    history of, 243–244
    special issues for, 250–252
    training in, 245–249
Psychopharmacology
    addiction psychiatry and, 231
    career opportunities in, 25, 27–29
    economics of, 31–32
    geriatric psychiatry and, 199
    history of, 25–27
    legal issues in, 32
    specific study populations and, 32–33
    training programs in, 29–31
Psychosomatic disorders, consultation-liaison psychiatry and, 77, 79

Publication, of research results, 9

Race. *See* Minorities
Rapid eye movement (REM) sleep, 35–36, 37
Relationship problems
  in student psychiatric population, 115–116
  group therapy and, 262–263
Research, psychiatric
  academic psychiatry and, 163–164
  addiction psychiatry and, 232
  administrative psychiatry and, 172, 178–179
  attributes of successful researcher, 5–9, 21–24
  career opportunities in, 3–5
  case study approach to careers in, 17–21
  child psychiatry and, 189–190
  on dreaming, 37–38
  forensic psychiatry and, 223
  on mental health aspects of reproductive function, 86
  in occupational psychiatry, 105–106
  in psychopharmacology, 27, 31–32, 32–33
  training for careers in, 9–14, 17–18, 23
Residencies. *See also* Training programs
  in administrative psychiatry, 175
  in educational psychiatry, 118
Rural areas
  administrative duties of psychiatrists in, 172
  emergency psychiatry in, 68
  private practice in, 94

Schedules, work
  in educational psychiatry, 120–121
  in emergency psychiatry, 71
Self-esteem, occupational psychiatry and, 104–105
Self-help groups, addiction psychiatry and, 230–231, 236
Setting-related careers
  in academic psychiatry, 157–167
  in community psychiatry, 133–140
  in consultation-liaison psychiatry, 77–86
  in educational psychiatry, 113–122
  in emergency psychiatry, 65–74
  in health maintenance organization psychiatry, 125–131
  in inpatient psychiatry, 51–62
  in military psychiatry, 143–153

Index

in occupational psychiatry, 103–110
in private practice, 91–101
Sleep disorders medicine
  advantages and disadvantages of careers in, 40–41
  duties of specialists in, 38–40
  economics of, 43–44
  education in, 41–42
  history of, 35–36
  legal issues in, 44–45
  professional organizations in, 42–43
  and psychiatry today, 37–38
Sleep Research Society (SRS), 43
Somnology. *See* Sleep disorders medicine
Specialty areas, careers in
  academic psychiatry, 157–158
  administrative psychiatry, 176–179
  child psychiatry, 185–194
  forensic psychiatry, 211–224
  geriatric psychiatry, 197–208
Staff-model health maintenance organizations, 126
State hospitals. *See also* Mental hospitals
  elderly in patient populations of, 207
  inpatient psychiatry in, 56–57
  psychopharmacology in, 27–28
Stress, occupational psychiatry and, 109
Student Mental Health Services. *See* Educational psychiatry
Suicide
  consultation psychiatry and, 82
  educational psychiatry and, 116
System design, community psychiatrists and, 138–139

Teaching, career opportunities in
  academic psychiatry, 161–163
  educational psychiatry, 118
  forensic psychiatry, 224
  military psychiatry, 148
  occupational psychiatry, 105–106
Telemedicine space bridge, 144, 148
Tort litigation, 215
Trainees, educational psychiatry and supervision of, 118
Training analyst, 250
Training programs
  for addiction psychiatry, 235
  for administrative psychiatry, 174–176
  for child psychiatry, 189
  for consultation-liaison psychiatry, 80–81

Training programs *(continued)*
  for emergency psychiatry, 71–72
  for family therapy, 257–259
  for forensic psychiatry, 214–215
  for geriatric psychiatry, 201–203
  for group therapy, 264–265
  for military psychiatry, 150
  for occupational psychiatry, 109–110
  for psychoanalysis, 245–249
  for psychopharmacology, 29–31
  for private practice, 97
  for psychiatrist-researchers, 9–14, 17–18, 23
Transference
  educational psychiatry and, 118
  psychoanalysis and, 244–245
Treatment modalities, careers based on
  family therapy, 255–259
  group therapy, 261–267
  psychoanalysis, 243–252

Uniformed Services University of the Health Sciences (USUHS) School of Medicine, 148
Universities. *See* Academic psychiatry; Educational psychiatry; Medical schools; Teaching
Utilization reviews, 125–126

Values. *See also* Ethics
  of psychiatrist-researcher, 9
  research training programs and institutional, 11–12
Vendors, in occupational medicine, 108
Veterans Administration
  addiction psychiatry and, 235
  geriatric psychiatry and, 202, 205
Violence, forensic psychiatry and, 222

Win–win approach, to conflict resolution, 174
Women, career opportunities for
  in academic psychiatry, 165–166
  in addiction psychiatry, 236–237
  in administrative psychiatry, 179–180
  in child psychiatry, 193–194
  in consultation-liaison psychiatry, 85
  in geriatric psychiatry, 207
  in military psychiatry, 151
  in private practice, 95
  in psychoanalysis, 251–252
Workers' compensation, 216